Social (In)Justice and Mental Health

Social (In)Justice and Mental Health

Edited by

Ruth S. Shim, M.D., M.P.H.
Sarah Y. Vinson, M.D.

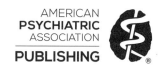

AMERICAN
PSYCHIATRIC
ASSOCIATION

PUBLISHING

If you wish to buy 50 or more copies of the same title, please go to www.appi.org/specialdiscounts for more information.

Copyright © 2021 American Psychiatric Association Publishing
ALL RIGHTS RESERVED
First Edition
Manufactured in the United States of America on acid-free paper
24 23 22 21 20   5 4 3 2 1
American Psychiatric Association Publishing
800 Maine Avenue SW
Suite 900
Washington, DC 20024-2812
www.appi.org

Library of Congress Cataloging-in-Publication Data
Names: Shim, Ruth S., 1977– editor. | Vinson, Sarah Y., editor. | American Psychiatric Association Publishing, publisher.
Title: Social (in)justice and mental health / edited by Ruth S. Shim, Sarah Y. Vinson.
Other titles: Social injustice and mental health
Description: First edition. | Washington, DC : American Psychiatric Association Publishing, [2021] | Includes bibliographical references and index.
Identifiers: LCCN 2020046148 (print) | LCCN 2020046149 (ebook) | ISBN 9781615373383 (paperback ; alk. paper) | ISBN 9781615373765 (ebook)
Subjects: MESH: Mental Health | Socioeconomic Factors | Health Equity | Mental Disorders | United States
Classification: LCC RA418 (print) | LCC RA418 (ebook) | NLM WM 31 | DDC 362.1—dc23
LC record available at https://lccn.loc.gov/2020046148
LC ebook record available at https://lccn.loc.gov/2020046149

British Library Cataloguing in Publication Data
A CIP record is available from the British Library.

In memory of Carl Compton Bell, M.D.
A prolific scholar, dedicated clinician, and fearless advocate—
the quintessential social justice psychiatrist

Contents

Part I

FOUNDATIONS OF SOCIAL INJUSTICE

Part II

SYSTEMS AND STRUCTURES

Part III

DIAGNOSES AND CONDITIONS

Part IV

ACHIEVING MENTAL HEALTH EQUITY

Contributors

Seyi O. Amosu, Ph.D.
Postdoctoral Fellow, Counseling Center, Georgia State University, Atlanta, Georgia

Deidre M. Anglin, Ph.D.
Associate Professor of Clinical Psychology, Department of Psychology, Graduate Center, City College of the City University of New York, New York, New York

Belinda Bandstra, M.D., M.A.
Assistant Director of Residency Training and Clinical Associate Professor, Department of Psychiatry and Behavioral Sciences, Stanford University School of Medicine, Stanford, California

Nicolás E. Barceló, M.D.
Postdoctoral Felllow, National Clinician Scholars Program, University of California, Los Angeles, Los Angeles, California

Khalima A. Bolden, Ph.D.
Licensed Clinical Psychologist, Assistant Director of Clinical Training, Davis Medical Center Early Psychosis Program, University of California, Davis, Sacramento, California

Brennin Y. Brown, M.D.
Psychiatry Resident, Case Western Reserve University, University Hospitals Cleveland Medical Center, Cleveland, Ohio

Melissa D. Carter, J.D.
Clinical Professor of Law and Executive Director of the Barton Child Law and Policy Center, Emory Law School, Atlanta, Georgia

Roy Collins, M.D., M.P.H.
Resident, Department of Psychiatry and Behavioral Sciences, Stanford University School of Medicine, Stanford, California

Michael T. Compton, M.D., M.P.H.
Professor of Psychiatry, Columbia University Vagelos College of Physicians and Surgeons, New York State Psychiatric Institute, New York, New York

Nicole Cotton, M.D.
Assistant Professor of Psychiatry, Morehouse School of Medicine, Atlanta, Georgia

Angie Lisbeth Cruz, M.H.S.
Ph.D. student, Department of Health Policy and Management, Rollins School of Public Health at Emory University, Atlanta, Georgia

Janet R. Cummings, Ph.D.
Associate Professor, Department of Health Policy and Management, Rollins School of Public Health at Emory University, Atlanta, Georgia

Kali D. Cyrus, M.D., M.P.H.
Assistant Professor, Department of Psychiatry and Behavioral Science, Johns Hopkins University School of Medicine, Baltimore, Maryland

Matthew L. Edwards, M.D.
Chief Resident, Department of Psychiatry and Behavioral Sciences, Stanford University School of Medicine, Stanford, California

David Freedman, Ph.D.
Senior Research Consultant, International Academy of Law and Mental Health, New York, New York

Mindy Thompson Fullilove, M.D.
Professor of Urban Policy and Health, Milano School of Public Policy, Management, and Environment, The New School, New York, New York

Poh Choo How, M.D., Ph.D.
Assistant Clinical Professor, Department of Psychiatry and Behavioral Sciences, University of California, Davis, Sacramento, California

Jessica Isom, M.D., M.P.H.
Attending Psychiatrist, Codman Square Health Center, Boston, Massachusetts

Jacob Michael Izenberg, M.D.
Clinical Assistant Professor, Department of Psychiatry, University of California, San Francisco, San Francisco, California

Michelle Ko, M.D., Ph.D.
Assistant Professor, Division of Health Policy and Management, Department of Public Health Sciences, University of California, Davis, Davis, California

Tiffani Marie, Ph.D.
Postdoctoral Fellow, Community Responsive Education, San Francisco, California

Courtney L. McMickens, M.D., M.P.H., M.H.S.
Psychiatrist, Cityblock Health, Inc., Brooklyn, New York

Phillip Murray, M.D., M.P.H.
Assistant Professor of Psychiatry, Atrium Health, Charlotte, North Carolina

Swati Rao, M.D.
Assistant Clinical Professor, Department of Psychiatry and Behavioral Sciences, University of California, Davis, Sacramento, California

LeRoy E. Reese, Ph.D.
Associate Professor of Community Health and Preventive Medicine, Kennedy Satcher Center for Mental Health Equity, Morehouse School of Medicine, Atlanta, Georgia

Samuel Ricardo Saenz, M.D., M.P.H.
Resident, Department of Psychiatry and Behavioral Sciences, Stanford University School of Medicine, Stanford, California

Sonya M. Shadravan, M.D.
Clinical and Forensic Psychiatrist, Office of Diversion and Reentry, Los Angeles, California

Ruth S. Shim, M.D., M.P.H.
Luke and Grace Kim Professor in Cultural Psychiatry and Professor, Department of Psychiatry and Behavioral Sciences, University of California, Davis, Sacramento, California

Sarah Y. Vinson, M.D.
Founder and Principal Consultant, Lorio Forensics; Associate Professor of Psychiatry and Pediatrics, Morehouse School of Medicine, Atlanta, Georgia

Melvin Wilson, M.B.A., L.C.S.W.
Senior Policy Consultant, Social Justice and Human Rights, National Association of Social Workers, Washington, DC

Walter E. Wilson Jr., M.D., M.H.A.
Child and Adolescent Psychiatry Fellow, Vanderbilt University Medical Center, Nashville, Tennessee

George W. Woods, M.D., LFAPA
University of California–Berkeley School of Law, Berkeley, California

Disclosure of Interests

The following contributors to this book have indicated a financial interest in or other affiliation with a commercial supporter, a manufacturer of a commercial product, a provider of a commercial service, a nongovernmental organization, and/or a government agency, as listed below:

Kali D. Cyrus, M.D., M.P.H.   *Honorarium*, Time's UP Healthcare speaking engagements
Ruth S. Shim, M.D., M.P.H.   *Member*, Board of Trustees, Robert Wood Johnson Foundation
Sarah Y. Vinson, M.D.   *Owner*, Lorio Psych group, consultation company that provides psychiatric services; Medical Advisory Group for Amerigroup Georgia

The following contributors have indicated that they have no financial interests or other affiliations that represent or could appear to represent a competing interferes with their contributions to this book:

Seyi O. Amosu, Ph.D.; Deidre M. Anglin, Ph.D.; Belinda Bandstra, M.D., M.A.; Nicolás E. Barceló, M.D.; Khalima A. Bolden, Ph.D.; Brennin Y. Brown, M.D.; Melissa D. Carter, J.D.; Roy Collins, M.D., M.P.H.; Michael T. Compton, M.D.; M.P.H.; Nicole Cotton, M.D.; Angie Lisbeth Cruz, M.H.S.; Janet R. Cummings, Ph.D.; Matthew L. Edwards, M.D.; David Freedman, Ph.D.; Mindy Thompson Fullilove, M.D.; Poh Choo How, M.D., Ph.D.; Jessica Isom, M.D., M.P.H.; Jacob Michael Izenberg, M.D.; Michelle Ko, M.D., Ph.D.; Tiffani Marie, Ph.D.; Phillip Murray, M.D.; M.P.H.; Swati Rao, M.D.; LeRoy E. Reese, Ph.D.; Samuel Ricardo Saenz, M.D., M.P.H.; Sonya M. Shadravan, M.D.; Ruth S. Shim, M.D., M.P.H.; Walter E. Wilson Jr., M.D., M.H.A.; George W. Woods, M.D., LFAPA

Foreword

I am a general pediatrician, not a mental health specialist. So why am I writing the foreword to a book about mental health and not children's health? In part because I am head of the Robert Wood Johnson Foundation, and our focus is on health equity. Also because the issues of social injustice are relevant to all areas of health. I've been taking care of children for more than 30 years, always in the setting of community clinics, providing services for children on Medicaid or without any health insurance at all. Over the course of my career, my perspective on health and my role as a physician has changed dramatically. Early on, I focused primarily on the list of items I was expected to cover at each well-child check: nutritional assessment, developmental assessment, various types of screening, and, of course, immunizations. I knew the guidelines from the American Academy of Pediatrics and the Centers for Disease Control and Prevention inside and out. My questions focused on teaching parents and children about health and healthy behaviors.

"Where does your baby sleep? It is important to put your baby on his back to sleep. That can reduce the chances of sudden infant death syndrome."

"What are you feeding your baby? Breastfeeding is best."

"What does she like to drink? Sugar-sweetened beverages are empty calories."

"How many hours is he sleeping? Sleep is critical. "

"How much screen time does she get? The Academy recommends no more than 2 hours per day."

"Let's talk about physical exercise. The CDC recommends 1 hour a day. How many hours does your child get?"

I'd march through the questions, document the answers in the electronic medical record, and order age-appropriate tests and vaccinations. Mission accomplished. Yet something about these interactions felt unsettling. So many of my patients and their families were struggling, and the issues that concerned them were not always physical ailments. Instead, the issues were the broader challenges in their lives. I was their doctor, but I wasn't dealing with the full picture of their well-being.

When I began working at the Robert Wood Johnson Foundation, I learned much more about the deeply rooted structural barriers that were impacting my patients' physical and mental health. And I had to ask myself a difficult question: Was the way I was delivering care part of the problem? The painful answer was "yes." I had to take a hard look at the assumptions and biases I was carrying into the clinic with me. I had to slow down. Ask more, and different, questions. And really listen. Then my understanding started to change.

I remember a conversation with a grandmother in Harlem. She was caring for her two grandsons, ages 9 and 11. I asked about physical activity, and she told me that her kids got only about 30 minutes of exercise twice a week, in school. I started to tell her about the CDC guidelines, and she stopped me. "I know that," she said. "But it's not safe for them to be outside playing in our neighborhood."

There was another conversation with a mother whose toddler son had asthma. We had been trying different approaches with medications, but he still kept ending up in the emergency department. Her son was allergic to dust mites, and as we continued to talk, I learned they lived in an apartment plagued with them. She had asked her landlord repeatedly to do a deep clean and make the place safe. But he was unwilling, and she didn't have the resources to do it herself or to move.

As health care workers, it's impossible for us to divorce our work from the relentless societal challenges our patients face. We have to expand our field of intervention beyond the consultation room. To have care about the conditions of the communities in which our patients live. And we have to weigh the impact that unfair policies have on their opportunity to thrive. Otherwise, we're not getting to the heart of the matter; we're just nibbling around the edges, and our treatment plans will continue to fall short.

I live in Princeton, New Jersey. It's the town I grew up in, and it is also the home of the Robert Wood Johnson Foundation, where I work. Life expectancy for a child born in this largely white, affluent community is 87 years. It has some of the best schools in the nation, secure neighborhoods, and ample green space for outdoor activities. I volunteer in a medical clinic just 14 miles away, in Trenton, New Jersey. These two cities are in the same county, but they might as well be on different planets. Trenton is not affluent, the population is mostly Black, and the life expectancy for a child born near the medical clinic is 73 years. That's a difference of 14 years in 14 miles. I think about that every time I make the drive. The families who live in Trenton and Princeton all care about their health and well-being. They have the same dreams and aspirations for their children. They work hard and strive to prosper. So how is it that one community can provide so much opportunity for health, while another just down the road makes it so much harder?

We like to think of America as the land of opportunity, but that opportunity isn't distributed fairly, and that is why social justice is a health issue. Access to jobs that pay a living wage is a health issue. Transportation is a health issue. Our nation's long history of racism and intentional segregation is a health issue. And the ongoing legacy of prejudicial policies that have kept families of color from building generational wealth is a health issue.

This book, *Social (In)Justice and Mental Health*, stresses the indisputable connection between equity and well-being. The authors recount how racism and other forms of injustice have contaminated the mental health profession, from the biased development of criteria for various diagnoses to the inequitable ways that patients are treated. The authors argue strongly and convincingly for a new approach to mental health care—one that acknowledges social injustice as a root cause of mental suffering. And most important, they offer individuals in the profession a path toward positive change.

I'm writing this foreword in the year 2020, when the critical need for structural change throughout every segment of our health care system has been laid bare. The unprecedented confluence of a viral pandemic, economic devastation, and a nationwide antiracism movement this year has revealed profoundly devastating fissures in our society, with Black, Latinx, and Indigenous people suffering and dying from illness, police violence, and racism at rates that surpass their proportion of the population.

How will historians record the reckonings of 2020? What will they write about our responses? Will they say we recognized the connections between social justice and health? Will they say we consciously worked to dismantle unjust systems?

The authors of this book believe positive change is truly possible, and that is what makes their insights so powerful. What could our nation look like if every health care provider embraced working toward social justice as a fundamental part of their profession? I'd like to think historians will point to 2020 as a true inflection point in America's road toward health equity and social justice. This book is an important part of that journey. And for those of you in the field of mental health, you can start by turning the page.

Richard E. Besser, M.D.
President and CEO, Robert Wood Johnson Foundation

Prologue

November 2019

Our first round of edits for this book took place on a work retreat in San Miguel de Allende, a city in central Mexico named for General Ignacio Allende, a prominent figure in Mexico's War of Independence. The city is famous for its well-preserved colonial and Spanish architecture, so on one of our breaks, we took a guided Tacos and Tequila tour through the rolling cobblestone streets, around the tree-lined town square, and under the twinkling string lights. Despite San Miguel's namesake, the tour guide, a friendly Latinx man in his early twenties, defaulted to telling the city's story from the perspective of the Spanish conquerors rather than that of the oppressed Indigenous people or the victorious revolutionaries. After a few tequila stops and our repeated nudges to share the landmarks' real stories, he opened up not only about injustice in San Miguel de Allende but also about his personal experiences of injustice in the United States.

Although born in Mexico, he came to the U.S. with his family when he was very young. He grew up in Florida and Georgia and stayed clear of the authorities—until he was flagged as undocumented during a minor traffic stop. Unsure of whether he qualified for the Development, Relief, and Education for Alien Minors (DREAM) Act, and without the money for an immigration attorney, he had never pursued that path before his arrest. He was incarcerated immediately. The funds his family scraped together to pay an attorney were pocketed by the officer of the court who did nothing to help him.

After being jailed for over a year, our affable tour guide was deported—away from his family of origin—and returned to an unknown and unfamiliar country. Although he had some extended family in Mexico, the loss of his home and the trauma of his incarceration led to despair and self-medication with crystal methamphetamine. He spoke of his path to recovery and his family's reality in the United States; how fear of deportation and mistreatment by those in authority relegated his loved ones to going straight from work or school to home; how their lives were defined by work, constricted by the need to lay low, and shaped by fear of detention and deportation. He openly shared that despite his path and the uphill battle he faced after his forced relocation to Mexico, he was happier now because he felt mentally freed. As two so-called experts, we were humbled by what our guide taught us about the power of perspective. We left San Miguel de Allende with a renewed appreciation for the humanity of the people we often overlook and for the direct impact that society's choices have on the mental well-being of these individuals.

May 2020

Our last round of edits for this book took place on our home soil as we, two Black women in opposite corners of the United States (California and Georgia), watched the most dramatic manifestations of the devaluations of Black lives in our lifetimes. Coronavirus disease 2019 (COVID-19), with its first U.S. case in northern California, laid bare the deadly implications of chronic, intergenerational health, employment, and socioeconomic racial inequities, exacting an age-adjusted death rate for Black people at 3.6 times that for white people. Meanwhile, the shooting death of Ahmaud Arbery in Georgia bubbled beneath the national consciousness until the nation watched George Floyd die with a police officer's knee on his neck. The two men's names became part of a tragic trio, also including that of first re-sponder Breonna Taylor, who was killed by police while asleep in her home, bound together in protest chants of "Say Their Names." The killing of George Floyd broadcast to a world slowed by COVID-19, imprinting on the American psyche the words first made famous by another unarmed Black man killed by police, Eric Garner: "I can't breathe."

COVID-19 is literally taking people's breath away. So, too, is the killing of unarmed Black people. Injustice and oppression take lives. And they shape them. An understanding of social injustice must inform every aspect of how we think about mental health and substance use disorders, their di-agnosis, and their treatment. We edited and finalized this book in equal measure tired, afraid—and resolute. We are frankly fed up with every sys-tem, including our own, that perpetuates rather than fights injustice. We humbly hope that *Social (In)Justice and Mental Health* becomes part of the arsenal for mental health professionals who understand that without justice there can be no peace.

Sarah Y. Vinson, M.D.
Atlanta, Georgia

Ruth S. Shim, M.D., M.P.H.
Sacramento, California

Preface

> I love America more than any other country in the world,
> and, exactly for this reason, I insist on the right to criticize
> her perpetually.
>
> *James Baldwin*, Notes of a Native Son

For the two of us, psychiatry is not merely a chosen specialty, a career, or even a profession—it is a calling. We are privileged and grateful to contribute in some small part to the dynamic, multifaceted, exciting field of mental health—a field in which relationships change lives. For two Black women psychiatrists in an occupation in which only 2% are Black, this privilege is even more profound. We hold the mental health profession in high esteem. We know how much it matters to our colleagues, our patients, and our larger society.

It is for this reason that we insist on viewing the field with an unflinchingly critical eye. It is for this reason that this book's content is informed by data rather than by sentiment. And it is for this reason that we concluded that this book could not be named *Social Justice and Mental Health* as we had originally planned. In compiling this book, the recurring theme throughout the research, editing, and revision process was one not of justice but of injustice. While it is true that inequities in mental health are complex, are deeply entrenched, and have multiple drivers, it is also true that society's pervasive injustices permeate our field, our diagnoses, and our systems. Our profession, shaped and practiced in the context of oppression, also plays a major role in perpetuating and sustaining inequity. Our relentless focus on individual pathology relegates social injustices to the periphery of our diagnostic formulations. However, on the basis of society's declining mental health status and consistently poor outcomes for many, our current approach has not been effective.

The authors of this book endeavor to introduce many readers to the concept of social justice and the outsized, but often ignored, role that social injustice plays in the identification, diagnosis, and management of mental illnesses and substance use disorders. Social injustice sustains mental health disparities and inequities, leads to reliably poor outcomes for highly treatable illnesses, and limits the potential for recovery.

Many great minds have attempted to solve the issue of mental health disparities in the United States. Highly intelligent, multidisciplinary teams of experts have come together to examine the literature, determining that patient-, provider-, and systems-level factors lead to disparities in health outcomes. Professionals in the mental health field have attempted to tackle this problem head-on, with significant focus on trying to address what can be more readily changed: patient- and provider-level factors. These efforts have led to training mental health professionals to be culturally competent, educating patients to reduce their stigma about mental illnesses, and encouraging patients to access care. There has been significant progress in these areas, yet mental health disparities and inequities persist. As professionals and as a society, we have neglected to tackle systems-level barriers with the same fervor and intensity as patient- and provider-level factors. It is time to examine the structures and systems that are driving mental health disparities and inequities.

This book is divided into four parts. In Part I, we define the foundational elements and theories of social injustice. In Part II, we describe the role of systems and structures and how they interact with mental health. In Part III, we discuss specific mental health conditions and diagnoses, reanalyzed through a social justice lens. Finally, Part IV is a guide on how to take action to achieve mental health equity. Of note, the various categorizations for people used in this book are reflective of contemporary academic and journalistic practice and the publisher's conventions. However, they do not necessarily reflect how members of these groups would categorize themselves. Furthermore, these categories are neither static nor precise. With time, and as a more representative group of those being defined become definers, it is anticipated that understanding will evolve and, in turn, so will the terminology for these categorizations.

We anticipate that this book will affect readers in different ways. Some of you have been on the front lines and in the trenches, doing the hard work for quite some time. You have championed issues of social justice throughout your careers and have dared to speak out against injustice, many times at risk to your own professional aspirations. You have inspired us to continue when things became difficult. We are honored to be members of this shared, supportive, and courageous community. Consider this book our thank you note for your work—we acknowledge the sacrifices you have made to advance mental health equity and we hope this book provides you with a scholarly resource to help support your ongoing efforts.

Some readers will find aspects of this book challenging because of their personal, lived experiences (past and present) with structural violence and social injustice. For these readers, we hope that our attempts to shine a light on a neglected area in mental health do not lead to vicarious harm.

Please prioritize your well-being with multiple check-ins and a focus on self-care as you read this book.

Other readers of this book will struggle with the content. These are difficult and uncomfortable topics. The discussion of these issues stirs up many emotions, including sadness, guilt, anger, fear, and resentment. You may perceive us to be accusing you of some of the behaviors described in the book, including racism, classism, sexism, ableism, homophobia, transphobia, xenophobia, and others. You may perceive us—especially as two Black women psychiatrists—as having a specific political agenda and lacking in objectivity. We have faced harsh, irrational, and even racist criticism before. But the issues delineated in this book are not going away. As mental health professionals, we have a responsibility to face, explore, and examine complicated emotions—in our patients and in ourselves. Complex emotions may arise for those who have never considered these topics before, for those who have considered them with alternative theoretical frames from those contained herein, and even for those who have been championing these issues for decades. If you happen to notice some of these negative emotions rising in you, please take a moment to stop, take a deep breath, and practice self-reflection. Be willing to sit with and explore the emotion for a bit. *It is an opportunity for growth.*

Often, as mental health professionals who support patients in confronting hard truths about their past, themselves, and their relationships with others, we tell our patients that they may feel worse before they feel better. This is because we know that confrontation, while necessary for healing, is hard. We know that uncomfortable truths that are tucked neatly away and compartmentalized impair functioning. As mental health professionals, we acknowledge that therapy is challenging, but we insist that it is worth it because the process will leave our patients more insightful and better able to build the lives they desire.

To our valued colleagues, for many of you, this content will be similarly challenging. Confronting hard truths about our profession's past and present, while demanding, is needed for us to do this vitally necessary work. In the words of James Baldwin, "Ignorance, allied with power, is the most ferocious enemy justice can have." As mental health professionals, we enjoy many forms of privilege—our income, education, and titles, to name a few. Our work and our approach can shape life trajectories. Our assessments, diagnoses, treatments, and administrative choices hold power. For far too long, we have wielded this power ignorant to the oppressive context that weighs on the backs of our patients' lives. Our ability to heal has been impaired.

So, in recognition that the content will be challenging for some because it contradicts current beliefs, we offer a few guidelines for how to go about reading this book. First and foremost, please consider reading with an open mind and an open heart. Consider the personal perspectives and the lifetime of experiences that you bring to your profession. And consider—as difficult as it may be—that the frame of your worldview may be flawed because these structural inequities are so ingrained in our society that they have essentially been rendered invisible. With this book, we aim to make the invisible visible. However, there must be an openness to receiving this information in order to see that which is not readily apparent and that is in conflict with what you sincerely believe to be true.

We encourage all who engage with this book to do so at a slow pace. As we have discussed, the content requires self-reflection, and progress from self-reflection takes time and effort. Our expert authors have taken great pains to make the content as readable, scholarly, and thoroughly honest as possible. By design, the chapters are relatively short so that a chapter can be read in one sitting, followed by ample time to reflect on the reading. To help guide your reading, we have included three self-reflection questions at the end of each chapter. Take the time to consider them. To that end, it might be helpful to read this book with other people and to dialogue about the content with other mental health professionals who both share and disagree with your perspectives.

We are indebted to our chapter authors, who contributed to this work beyond measure with their perspectives, their expertise, and their fearlessness in expressing truth, anchored in deeply intellectual thought. Additionally, this work could not have been accomplished without the loving support of our families and friends, the guidance and wisdom of our mentors, and the energy and creativity of our students and trainees. But most importantly, this book would not exist if not for our many patients, past and present, who have taught us so much about dignity, resilience, and courage in the face of insurmountable obstacles in their lives. They are our inspiration and the reason why we cannot fail in our task.

As the editors of this book, and more importantly, as your colleagues who are privileged to do this work, we have prioritized the examination of hard truths about our practice, our profession, and our society over the employment of euphemisms or strategic omissions in the hopes of striking a more optimistic tone. Rather, this book's critical and, at times, righteously angry tone is rooted in something much more important: the optimistic belief that all of us hold untapped potential to advance mental health equity and the genuine hope that, collectively, we can make meaningful progress toward this goal.

Sarah Y. Vinson, M.D.
Atlanta, Georgia

Ruth S. Shim, M.D., M.P.H.
Sacramento, California
May 2020

PART I
FOUNDATIONS OF SOCIAL INJUSTICE

CHAPTER 1

Social (In)Justice and Mental Health

Ruth S. Shim, M.D., M.P.H.
Sarah Y. Vinson, M.D.

What Is Social Justice?

Extensive debate about the meaning and intent of the term *social justice* persists, despite its having deep roots in contemporary philosophy. Like many things that are associated with politics, the definition and use of the term have been distorted and misrepresented over time. On a basic level, however, the concept is quite simple. American philosopher John Rawls (2003) defined social justice as "assuring the protection of equal access to liberties, rights, and opportunities, as well as taking care of the least advantaged members of society" (Robinson 2010, p. 79). When stated this way, the principles of social justice seem like values that everyone can support.

Yet in some circles, social justice has a bad reputation. The term *social justice warrior*, added to the *Oxford English Dictionary* in 2015, is used pejoratively to describe people who espouse values of feminism, civil rights, and social progressivism. Recently, physicians and others have expressed criticism of the growing role of social justice in medicine, as exemplified by a high-profile op-ed published in the *Wall Street Journal* (Goldfarb 2019).

Doctors and other health professionals have been encouraged to "stay in their lane." Despite this criticism, social justice is still considered to be the moral foundation of public health. In fact, the American Public Health Association (2020) asserts that structured inequities "sap our potential to become the healthiest nation."

This book, however, is not about social justice. This book is about social *injustice*. The United States does not assure "the protection of equal access to liberties, rights, and opportunities" to everyone and does not excel in "taking care of the least advantaged members of society," to use the words of Rawls (2003). A perfect storm of unfair and unjust policies and practices, bolstered by deep-seated beliefs about the inferiority of some groups, has led to a small number of people in the United States having tremendous advantages, freedoms, and opportunities, while a growing number of people in the United States are denied liberties, human rights, and opportunities. As a society, we have received—sometimes covertly, sometimes overtly—inadequate explanations as to why this is the case. We are taught to believe in the "American Dream"—that all Americans have the opportunity to succeed if they have enough drive and ingenuity. This dream was founded on the concept of a *meritocracy* that espouses talent and drive as more important than money and class. However, the American Dream was founded on a lie, one that elevated white men above (and at the expense of) all other groups and ensured that they had *the most* advantages, liberties, rights, and opportunities. This belief in the superiority of white men when compared with other groups has invaded every aspect of American society, including medicine. In fact, this belief has infected the way we think about, diagnose, and treat mental illnesses.

As the authors explore in this book, our frames for determining what is normal and what is psychopathology are specifically filtered through a lens that has been distorted by social injustice. Why else do we so easily blame individuals for the challenges that they face in trying to live healthy, productive lives? And why else do we focus so singularly on the role of personal responsibility and free will in the pursuit of health?

Social Injustice and Mental Illnesses

Social injustice drives both mental illnesses and mental health inequities. Therefore, any discussion of either topic is incomplete without a deeper examination of the connection between social injustice and mental health. Where people live, work, and play has implications for how they think, feel, and behave, and these aspects of people's lives are influenced, at times even dictated, by social injustice. The varied forms of oppression that groups experience are mentally toxic forces and, when they are perpetuated by societal systems, are profoundly harmful. Every major U.S. system has been created and reformed in the context of social injustice and has, in turn, produced inequitable outcomes. The mental health system is no exception. Mental health professionals may not have personally borne the weight of these forces or may have been privileged to advance in their professions in spite of them. As a result, despite the ubiquity of its manifestations, social injustice is frequently glossed over or rationalized away by many mental health professionals.

Progress in medicine and mental health has led to the understanding that *nature versus nurture* is a false dichotomy and that it is the interaction of the two that produces health or illness. The next step is to understand the scope of the nurture component. Family dynamics are important but so too are the dynamics of the larger society. Far beyond the cradle to the grave, the interplay of injustice and biological risk starts prenatally and extends through generations. It is no wonder that this results in mental illnesses that manifest differently and at disparate frequencies in oppressed people.

Instructional methods, theoretical paradigms, assessment approaches, and service delivery methods have not resulted in equitable outcomes for two primary reasons:

1. They are interdependent with unjust schooling, housing, carceral (criminal justice), employment, and financial systems
2. They are dependent on theoretical paradigms disproportionately created and advanced by people who have benefited from these injustices

Our methods, paradigms, approaches, and services are contaminated. To understand individual patients, we as mental health professionals must deepen our understanding of broader society. We must question not only how it has shaped our patients' personal experiences but also its influence on our professional perspectives and practices.

Applying a Social Justice Lens

In the 1990s, the United States entered the "decade of the brain." Amazing neuroscience advances were made in mental health—especially in understanding that mental illnesses are brain diseases. More recently, a push to integrate neuroscience into training and clinical practice has taken hold (Arbuckle et al. 2017). However, the initial formulations of the biopsychosocial model do not discount the role of the social environment in the shaping and development of healthy brains and in the creation of mental illness. In some ways, in shifting to a neuroscience frame, we as mental health professionals have forgotten the important role of social factors in the development of disease. If we discount the role of social factors in the development of mental illness, then we also discount the social determinants of mental health—the main cause of mental health inequities. It is impossible to even begin to explain the deep inequities in the United States as they relate to mental health outcomes without a fundamental understanding of the role that social injustice plays in the development and shaping of disease. Neuroscience is not irrelevant, but its contributions to social determinants of mental health and mental health inequities are minimal. Attempts to contemplate inequities through the lens of neuroscience lead us at best to consider the importance of epigenetics and at worst to advance a type of biological determinism that implies that different outcomes in populations are the result of underlying biological differences (Graves 2015).

Unfortunately, medicine has long erred on the side of biological determinism and a belief in the inherent inferiority of some groups. In a letter to a colleague in 1931, pathologist and oncologist Cornelius Rhoads described his Puerto Rican patients as

> beyond doubt the dirtiest, laziest, most degenerate and thievish race of men ever inhabiting this sphere. They are even lower than Italians.... I have done my best to further the process of extermination by killing off eight and transplanting cancer into several more. The latter has not resulted in any fatalities so far. The matter of consideration for the patients' welfare plays no role here—in fact all physicians take delight in the abuse and torture of the unfortunate subjects. (Rhoads C, November 1931, personal communication)

Rhoads went on to have an illustrious career in medicine and was featured on the cover of *Time* magazine. When the letter was first discovered in 1932, and again later, when the American Association for Cancer Research stripped his name from a prestigious award, Rhoads had several defenders within the medical profession who asserted that the letter was a *joke* and "intended as a confidential note" (Rosenthal 2003). The fact that Rhoads was allowed to continue and have an illustrious career reflects the way medicine has repeatedly conferred advantages and benefits to some people even when doing so is in direct conflict with the well-being and safety of others.

Important Social Justice Concepts

Several concepts—oppression, implicit bias, privilege, othering, and intersectionality—require a basic level of understanding for readers to engage effectively with the work described in this book. As accomplished and smart professionals, we often feel we have a clear grasp of these concepts, but they are not routinely taught in standard medical educational paths. Thus, we define these important concepts so readers have a more universal comprehension of what is meant when the terms are used throughout the book.

Oppression

> Oppressive language does more than represent violence, it is violence; does more than represent the limits of knowledge, it limits knowledge.
>
> *Toni Morrison*

Oppression is a concept that is raised repeatedly throughout this book, yet it is not entirely well understood. Oppression is not routinely studied in medical school, graduate school, or mental health training and certificate programs. Political theorist Iris Marion Young (1990) described five types of oppression: exploitation, marginalization, powerlessness, cultural imperialism, and violence. Table 1–1 defines these types of oppression and provides examples of how they are expressed in mental health.

Unfortunately, in the United States, oppressed groups are too numerous to count. The goal of the authors of this book is to focus on evidence and data. Much of the data about the impact of oppression has focused on Black people, although some minimal data have been reported on Indigenous and Latinx people. The emphasis on Black people in this book may seem excessive, but it is reflective of the available evidence. We hope that this information and knowledge can be extrapolated and applied to other oppressed groups.

Implicit Bias

Implicit biases are the neurobiologically based attitudes that unconsciously affect one's decisions and behaviors. These biases are automatic and pervasive, and they can, at times, be in direct conflict with one's expressed beliefs or values (Staats et al. 2017). Because implicit bias is neurobiologically based, the goal is not to achieve a state in which one *has no bias*. Rather, the goal is to accept that one has biases, reflect on whether those biases are negative or positive, and endeavor to replace those negative biases that interfere with effective treatment of people with mental illnesses with more positive ones (Staats et al. 2017). Highly educated, logical scientists often struggle with this concept.

TABLE 1–1. Types of oppression and expressions in mental health

Type of oppression	Definition	Mental health expression
Exploitation	The unequal exchange of one group's labor and energies for another group's advantage and advancement	*Employment:* High rates of unemployment, underemployment, and job insecurity, coupled with weak social supports for job loss, lead to increased anxiety, depression, and substance misuse
Marginalization	Expelling of specific groups from meaningful participation in society	*Housing and the carceral (criminal justice) system:* Transinstitutionalization of people with serious mental illnesses leads to increased incarceration and homelessness
Powerlessness	Blocking specific groups from power and routes to gain power	*Education and income inequality:* Exclusion of oppressed groups from attaining higher education, high-level employment, and income; punishment of people in poverty through harsh requirements to receive and maintain social welfare support
Cultural imperialism	Establishment of the ruling class culture as the norm; othering of groups that are not part of the dominant culture	*Discrimination:* Implicit negative biases that imply that racial and ethnic minority groups are inferior; immigration policies that exclude or restrict entry of certain groups into the United States
Violence	Threats and experiences of physical and structural violence	*Exposure to violence:* People who are oppressed are at risk of experiencing domestic and interpersonal violence, as well as increased risk of being victims of hate crimes

Source.   Adapted from Young 1990.

Privilege

Outside of most people's conscious understanding, membership in certain social identity groups in the United States confers unearned benefits and advantages, which are referred to as *privileges*. Without self-reflection, it is difficult to recognize when one is the beneficiary of such advantage and easy to assume that these privileges are available to everyone. Most people, even people who are members of oppressed groups, have privileges in some aspects of society. The most important thing is how one chooses to use one's unearned privileges: in the service of seizing opportunities to advance oneself or to help those with fewer advantages? Although there is nothing inherently wrong with using unearned privileges to get ahead, privileges are a type of power that can be harnessed to address the structural inequities encountered in day-to-day experiences.

Othering

Othering is "a set of dynamics, processes, and structures that engender marginality and persistent inequality across any of the full range of human differences based on group identities" (powell and Menendian 2016, p. 17). It is based on the thought that a certain group threatens the existence and prosperity of one's own identified group. Fear of the other is a common strategy employed against marginalized populations, such as people with serious mental illnesses and substance use disorders, people with disabilities, transgender people, or people of color.

Intersectionality

Originally a legal term developed by Kimberlé Crenshaw (1990), *intersectionality* describes how different social group categorizations are interconnected, creating overlapping systems of oppression. For example, two groups that are highly oppressed in the United States are Black people and transgender people. However, intersectionality of these identities puts Black transgender and gender-nonconforming people at the highest risk of oppression in the form of violence as compared with all other groups. In 2019, of the 22 known victims of anti-transgender fatal violence in the United States, Black transgender women represented 91% of victims (Human Rights Campaign Foundation 2019).

Foundational Theories in Social Justice

Curiously, many Americans consider themselves to have expertise in issues of race and power, although they may have little by way of training, formal education, or self-study to support this belief. The authors of this book draw from an extensive body of research on social justice, including sociology, anthropology, critical ethnic studies, disability studies, Chicana/Chicano studies, Asian American studies, Black studies, American studies, Indigenous studies, gender studies, queer studies, critical race theory, liberation theology, and environmental studies, among others. The authors build on this immense foundation of scholarly thought because it is quite difficult to come to reasoned, scientifically accurate conclusions without the benefit of this prior knowledge. However, attempts to apply this foundation to the field of medicine and mental health has proven to be challenging in execution because most health professions educators do not have extensive knowledge in these disciplines.

The writer Chimamanda Ngozi Adichie (2009) talks about "the danger of a single story," in which power can allow people to tell one, limiting story about other groups of people. Indeed, in *A History of Psychiatry*, historian Edward Shorter (1997) paints an image of mental illness deeply influenced by European and white American ideals and thoughts in which Sigmund Freud and proponents of biological theories reign supreme. The result is a single story of the triumphs, successes, and occasionally failures of psychiatry—without an understanding of how bias, oppression, and structural forces intersect to create a skewed vision of mental health and illnesses in this country. If we neglect to understand the fullness of history, we miss an entire critical perspective, and we are then led to erroneous conclusions about the origins of disease. How can we tell the history of psychiatry without considering the impact of psychiatrist Frantz Fanon? How can we come to understand identity development without reflecting on the work of psychologist Mamie Clark? How can we contemplate teaching about culture and mental health without examining the writings of educator Paulo Freire? And how can we think about adverse childhood experiences without considering historical trauma as conceptualized by social worker Maria Yellow Horse Brave Heart? The single story we have been told is wholly inadequate, and as Toni Morrison said, "It limits knowledge."

Limitations of Social Justice Theory in Mental Health

There are some limitations to consider when contemplating the impact of social injustice on mental health. At a cursory glance, it may appear that we are attempting in this book to deemphasize biology and genetics. However, that is not our intention. Biology and genetics indeed play a role in the development of and outcomes associated with substance use disorders and other mental illnesses. It may seem that by choosing to focus on the social determinants of mental health, we are not acknowledging this role. Rather, we posit that the role of biology and genetics is relevant but not as infinitely relevant as we have been led to believe. According to studies of premature death rates (one of the best indicators of population health available), genetics contributes to about 30% of premature death; however, 70% of the determinants of premature death are attributable to environmental factors, behavioral patterns, social circumstances, and access to health care (McGinnis et al. 2002). These social determinants make up the majority of reasons for premature death, and they are intimately shaped by social injustice.

Another limitation of considering mental health inequities through a social justice frame is that it tends to minimize the importance of free will and personal responsibility. These are deeply held American ideals, and, yes, the choices we make contribute to the outcomes and differences in our health. However, the exercising of free will is constrained by oppression, structural discrimination, and social injustice. The statement "the choices we make are shaped by the choices we have" rings true here (California Newsreel 2008). Social injustice limits options and choices, effectively making personal responsibility less personal. Not everyone has the same options; some choose what they perceive to be the best choice from a range of disadvantageous choices.

Conclusion

The path to a mentally healthy society goes through justice. Just as mental health professionals must learn patients' history and functional impairments to effectively treat their symptoms, we also must learn (or, more accurately, re-learn) our society's history and structural injustices to effectively transform its systems. Even with time and great effort, some inequities may persist. Substantial progress toward mental health equity will not come overnight, and it will not come without struggle. In the absence of knowledge about social injustice, it is certain that mental health equity will not come at all.

Questions for Self-Reflection

1. What are my associations with social justice and/or social justice warriors? What are these associations based on?
2. Of the five types of oppression described, which am I least and most personally familiar with?
3. When I have experienced or witnessed oppression, how has it impacted my thoughts, feelings, or actions?

References

Adichie CN: The danger of a single story (video). New York, TED, July 2009. Available at: www.ted.com/talks/chimamanda_ngozi_adichie_the_danger_ of_a_single_story?language=en. Accessed May 10, 2020.

American Public Health Association: Social Justice and Health. Washington, DC, American Public Health Association, 2020. Available at: https://apha.org/what-is-public-health/generation-public-health/our-work/social-justice. Accessed May 3, 2020.

Arbuckle MR, Travis MJ, Ross DA: Integrating a neuroscience perspective into clinical psychiatry today. JAMA Psychiatry 74:313–314, 2017

California Newsreel: Unnatural Causes: Is Inequality Making us Sick? 10 Things to Know About Health. San Francisco, CA, 2008. Available at: https://unnatural causes.org/ten_things.php. Accessed September 5, 2020.

Crenshaw K: Mapping the margins: intersectionality, identity politics, and violence against women of color. Stanford Law Rev 43:1241–1299, 1990

Goldfarb S: Take two aspirin and call me by my pronouns. Wall Street Journal, September 12, 2019

Graves JL Jr: Great is their sin: biological determinism in the age of genomics. Ann Am Acad Pol Soc Sci 661:24–50, 2015

Human Rights Campaign Foundation: A National Epidemic: Fatal Anti-Transgender Violence in the United States in 2019. Washington, DC, Human Rights Campaign, November 2019. Available at: https://assets2.hrc.org/files/assets/resources/ Anti-TransViolenceReport2019.pdf?_ga=2.174642210.1837215665.1589077 647%E2%80%931126914729.1589077647. Accessed May 7, 2020.

McGinnis JM, Williams-Russo P, Knickman JR: The case for more active policy attention to health promotion. Health Aff 21:78–93, 2002

powell ja, Menendian S: The problem of othering. In Othering and Belonging: Expanding the Circle of Human Concern. Berkeley, CA, Haas Institute, 2016. Available at: www.otheringandbelonging.org/wp-content/uploads/2016/07/ OtheringAndBelonging_Issue1.pdf. Accessed June 24, 2020.

Rawls J: Justice as Fairness: Restatement, 2nd Edition. Boston, MA, Belknap, 2003

Robinson M: Assessing criminal justice practice using social justice theory. Soc Justice Res 23:77–97, 2010

Rosenthal ET: The Rhoads not given: the tainting of the Cornelius P. Rhoads Memorial Award. Oncology Times 25:19–20, 2003

Shorter E: A History of Psychiatry. New York, Wiley, 1997

Staats C, Capatosto K, Tenney L, Mamo S: State of the Science: Implicit Bias Review. Columbus, OH, Kirwan Institute for the Study of Race and Ethnicity, 2017

Young IM: Five faces of oppression, in Justice and the Politics of Difference. Princeton, NJ, Princeton University Press, 1990, pp 39–65

CHAPTER 2

Social Injustice and the Social Determinants of Mental Health

Ruth S. Shim, M.D., M.P.H.
Michael T. Compton, M.D., M.P.H.

In 2005, the World Health Organization convened the Commission on Social Determinants of Health, an international group of experts to marshal the best possible evidence to create a global movement to promote and achieve health equity. The Commission's final report, *Closing the Gap in a Generation: Health Equity Through Action on the Social Determinants of Health*, concluded that the "unequal distribution of health" was not a natural phenomenon and that it had no biological basis (Commission on Social Determinants of Health 2008). *Social determinants of health* are defined by the Commission as those "conditions in which people are born, grow, live,

The authors wish to acknowledge the helpful feedback and recommendations provided by Abdul Kamara, BVC, LLB, LLM.

work, and age," which are shaped by the distribution of money, power, and resources. Most importantly, the social determinants of health are a common cause of health inequities (World Health Organization 2020, p. 1).

There is little debate regarding the existence and persistence of mental health disparities and inequities. Extensive research has documented these differences in outcomes, including that racial and ethnic minority groups in the United States 1) have less access to and availability of care, 2) receive generally poorer quality of mental health services, and 3) experience a greater disability burden from unmet mental health needs (U.S. Department of Health and Human Services 2001). Considerable debate continues to exist, however, in regard to the primary causes of these mental health disparities and inequities. Routinely, disparities in mental health status among different populations are attributed to individual behavior, and specifically *how* individuals choose to interact with their environments. Many mental health professionals assume that racial and ethnic minority groups access care less frequently than majority groups because of cultural values and stigma about receiving mental health services. Some mental health professionals suggest that racial and ethnic minority groups receive poorer quality of mental health services because of workforce shortages and providers who are not effectively trained to interact with people who are different from them. And some mental health professionals propose that a greater disability burden comes from a lack of mental health literacy and education that leads to accessing services only when in crisis rather than before the problem has become unmanageable.

Many mental health professionals do not regularly consider the underlying factors that determine these differences in mental health outcomes. The drivers of these inequities, and true solutions for and progress toward eliminating them, have consistently remained out of reach. As a result, many mental health professionals provide care, run clinical services, and implement health policies while remaining unaware of the central role of social injustice in perpetuating health inequities. The United States holds strong to the values that individuals can make their own way in society and are the masters of their own destinies: If people are successful in life, it is because they worked harder and were smarter than others. If people fail or struggle, it could be because they are lazy and lack the desire or intellect to succeed. Therefore, it is not a great leap to erroneously conclude that if certain populations are more likely to suffer from the ill effects of mental illnesses and substance use disorders, it may be the result of group-level differences in biology and culture, coupled with individual-level choices. This is a very tempting stance to take because it absolves everyone (and mental health professionals in particular) from considering other, more structural factors contributing to poor mental health outcomes and inequities.

It is interesting to consider some common differences in mental health outcomes. Data that evaluate population groups on the basis of race, ethnicity, gender identity, or sexual orientation are quite complicated because these categories are all socially constructed; however, regardless of this imprecision, examination and interpretation of the available literature reveal interesting trends. Compared with men, women have a higher prevalence of eating disorders, depressive disorders, and anxiety disorders (Astbury 2001). Native Americans have a higher prevalence of alcohol use disorders compared with other racial groups (Chartier and Caetano 2010). Lesbian and bisexual women have higher rates of substance use disorders than do heterosexual women (Green and Feinstein 2012). Poor white and Indigenous young men are more likely than Black and Latinx young men to use crystal methamphetamine (Iritani et al. 2007). Adolescents with learning disabilities are more likely to develop a substance use disorder or a psychiatric disorder than are adolescents without learning disabilities (Beitchman et al. 2001). Transgender people are more likely than cisgender people to attempt suicide (Clements-Nolle et al. 2006). And individuals with serious mental illnesses (i.e., major depressive disorder, schizophrenia, and bipolar disorder) are more likely to die up to 25 years earlier than the general population (Parks et al. 2006). These outcomes are consistent and persistent over time.

These trends are traditionally considered to be *mental health disparities*, defined as differences in health status that occur among different population groups. The dominant narrative in medicine and medical education is that these are unavoidable differences that exist because of intrinsic (i.e., biological and cultural) differences. In reality, the differences described above are more accurately defined as *mental health inequities*—differences in health that are the result of *systemic, avoidable,* and *unjust* social and economic policies that create barriers to opportunity (Braverman 2016). Although there is a growing understanding of the role that the social determinants of health and mental health play in contributing to poor health outcomes, the mental health field has not consistently come to understand that many of these social determinants are the deliberate and inevitable result of structural forces that oppress and subjugate specific populations. In this chapter, we describe how the social determinants of mental health—the main causes of mental health inequities—are driven by social injustice in society.

The Social Determinants of Mental Health Framework

Social injustice is the foundation on which the social determinants of mental health are built. Figure 2–1 depicts a framework of the social determinants of mental health. Public policies and social norms (at the bottom of the figure) lead to the unequal and unjust distribution of opportunity, which in turn is expressed as social determinants of mental health. This unequal and unjust distribution of opportunity also interacts directly and indirectly with public policies and social norms, changing attitudes, perceptions, and actions taken to elevate and advantage some members of society while simultaneously working to oppress and disadvantage others. Inequitable distribution of opportunity leads to a host of pervasive, detrimental social problems, factors that bring about low socioeconomic status, unmet basic human needs, and immediate and global physical environmental threats. These social determinants of mental health are described in detail elsewhere (Compton and Shim 2015), but suffice it to say that ample data connect specific social determinants of mental health and poor mental health outcomes. Table 2–1 lists research examples for the social determinants of mental health specified in Figure 2–1.

Public policies are codes, rules, regulations, legislation, and court decisions about education, employment, wages, food, housing, neighborhoods, and many other facets of society. The laws and rules created and enforced in society that seemingly have no discernible connection to health often impart significant, lasting impacts on the health and well-being of the population. For example, the Social Security Act of 1935 created social security benefits for the aging population, a sweeping social protection policy that led to Americans being able to retire comfortably, build wealth, and pass financial gains on to future generations. This major public policy does not appear at first glance to be a health policy, but these investments in older adults helped to increase income, improve physical and mental health, and decrease mortality for their beneficiaries (Arno et al. 2011). Unfortunately, the discriminatory application of this policy, which initially excluded domestic and agricultural workers, most often Black and Latinx people, led to increased poverty and greater income inequality in these excluded populations, ultimately resulting in increased risk of physical and mental health problems and setting the stage for intergenerational poverty as well (DeWitt 2010). Thus, the differential application and enforcement of public policies against specific population groups also drive social injustice.

Since the founding of the United States, and with increasingly alarming intensity in recent years, federal public policies have been enacted to benefit a small, powerful elite group of people in society, most consistently including the top 1% of income earners. These individuals hold 40% of the U.S. share of wealth, which is more than the bottom 90% combined (Wolff 2017). In fact, 5.3 million American citizens live in absolute poverty conditions comparable to those of third-world countries (Alston 2018). Recent public policies, including federal tax cuts, have solely advantaged the rich

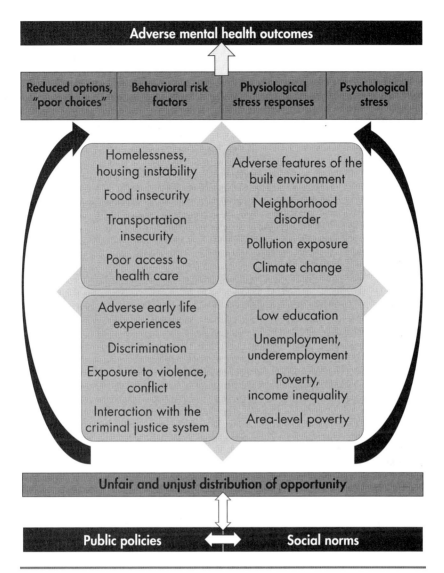

FIGURE 2–1.   Social determinants of mental health framework.
To view this figure in color, see Plate 1 in Color Gallery.

at the expense of the poor. Meanwhile, public policies have been enacted to eliminate social supports for the poorest and most vulnerable citizens of the United States. Proposals have been made to cut the Supplemental Nutrition Assistance Program, income assistance for people with disabilities, and housing and energy assistance (Parrott et al. 2018). These deliberate actions amplify the social injustices that lead to poor physical and mental health outcomes and widening health and mental health inequities.

TABLE 2–1.   Examples of associations between social
determinants and poor mental health
outcomes

Social determinant of mental health	Research example
Adverse early life experiences	There is a graded, dose-response relationship between the number of adverse childhood experiences and suicide attempts, alcohol use disorder, and substance misuse (Merrick et al. 2017)
Discrimination	Racism is associated with poorer mental health, including depression, anxiety, and psychological stress (Paradies et al. 2015)
Exposure to violence and conflict	Women who witnessed violent acts in their neighborhoods experience depressive and anxiety symptoms at twice the rate of women who did not witness community violence (Clark et al. 2008)
Interaction with the criminal justice system	Incarceration during adolescence and early adulthood is independently associated with increased depressive symptoms and suicidal thoughts in adulthood (Barnert et al. 2017)
Low education	School dropout at the elementary level is associated with higher risk of poor mental health compared with dropout at all other educational levels (Hjorth et al. 2016)
Unemployment and underemployment	Unemployment is strongly associated with increased alcohol and substance use disorders (Compton et al. 2014)
Poverty and income inequality	Countries with higher measures of income inequality have higher incidence of schizophrenia (Burns et al. 2014)
Area-level poverty	Childhood family poverty predicts PTSD and MDD diagnoses in adulthood (Nikulina et al. 2011)
Homelessness and housing instability	Unstable housing predicts depressive symptoms in people with substance use disorders (Davey-Rothwell et al. 2008)
Food insecurity	Food insecurity in young adults is associated with increased depression, suicidal ideation, and substance misuse (Pryor et al. 2016)
Transportation insecurity	Good access to public transportation reduces the risk of depression in women and older adults (Melis et al. 2015)
Poor access to health care	Individuals with Medicaid coverage have lower rates of depression than do those with no insurance (Baicker et al. 2013)

TABLE 2–1. Examples of associations between social determinants and poor mental health outcomes *(continued)*

Social determinant of mental health	Research example
Adverse features of the built environment	Higher levels of neighborhood green space are associated with lower levels of depression, anxiety, and stress (Beyer et al. 2014)
Neighborhood disorder	Neighborhood disadvantage is associated with higher rates of depression and substance use disorder (Silver et al. 2002)
Pollution exposure	High-resolution air pollution exposure at age 12 is associated with increased odds of major depressive disorder at age 18 (Roberts et al. 2019)
Climate change	Extreme weather events (e.g., storms, floods) are associated with higher rates of PTSD, particularly in developing countries (Rataj et al. 2016)

Note.   MDD=major depressive disorder; PTSD=posttraumatic stress disorder.

Social norms pertain to values, attitudes, impressions, and biases held by individuals in society and by the collective. Rather than being codified or officiated like public policies, social norms are largely learned and disseminated within groups. Instead of regulations, they are informal opinions and beliefs about people and social groups, including political ideologies as well as views on class, race and ethnicity, nationality, and gender, just to name a few. These social norms are deeply held beliefs that are ingrained in the fabric of society (Shim and Compton 2019). Of course, these beliefs can represent egregiously racist, classist, ableist, misogynistic, xenophobic, or any other overtly hateful thoughts, but more often, social norms are powered by implicit biases that are below the surface of awareness. These implicit beliefs are powerful mechanisms by which social norms lead to unfair and unjust distribution of opportunity and social determinants of mental health.

For example, the United States is a strongly patriarchal society, founded on principles that men are superior to women. As a result of these entrenched social norms, many people implicitly (and explicitly) believe that women are physically, intellectually, and temperamentally inferior to men. Inequitable social norms have led to violence and sexual trauma against women; a lack of women in science, technology, and medical fields; underrepresentation of women in positions of leadership; and societal acceptance of the routine nature of these injustices. Recent attempts to bring awareness to these issues, including the Me Too and Time's Up movements, may be subsiding over time as social norms revert to previous mindsets. Patriarchal social norms have led to the long-standing formal exclusion of women from political power and representation, which in turn lead to public policies that continue to reinforce these pernicious social norms. As a result, social norms about the inferiority of women impact all aspects of society, including failure to pass family leave policies, women's lack of representation in all levels of politics, and even the way that fundamental concepts of reproduction are taught in science courses (Martin 1991).

Unequal and Unjust Distribution of Opportunity

Harmful public policies and negative social norms lead to social injustice. The decisions that we collectively make as a society—who we value, who we oppress, who we believe is deserving of advantages, who we intentionally disadvantage in society—confer benefits to some groups at the expense of other groups. The unequal and unjust distribution of opportunity creates structural forces that lead to differential levels of harm in various communities and populations, a concept known as *structural violence*. This type of harm is so deeply embedded in the fabric of our society that it essentially becomes invisible (Farmer et al. 2006) and "may be seen as about as natural as the air around us" (Galtung 1969, p. 173).

The social determinants of mental health, then, are clear examples of structural violence because adverse childhood experiences, poverty, lack of access to health care, and low education directly lead to differential levels of harm, in the form of mental illnesses and substance use disorders. Also, because structural violence most specifically injures those groups that are oppressed, it also serves to exacerbate mental health inequities. Paulo Freire (1970) describes this type of harm as the result of "an unjust order that engenders violence in the oppressors, which in turn dehumanizes the oppressed" (p. 44). Indeed, oppression often presents itself in ways that are closely associated with poor outcomes associated with serious and persistent mental illnesses. As the Commission on Social Determinants of Health (2008) noted in *Closing the Gap in a Generation*, "Any serious effort to reduce health inequities will involve changing the distribution of power within society and global regions, empowering individuals and groups to represent strongly and effectively their needs and interests" (p. 18). Power dynamics in the United States ensure that privilege and resources are held by a very few, who often use this power to marginalize and exploit groups that do not hold power.

In 2018, a report by Philip Alston (2018), the special rapporteur on extreme poverty and human rights in the United States, was submitted to the United Nations Human Rights Council. Surprisingly, this report did not receive a great deal of public or political attention, but it highlighted the early mortality and increased risk of communicable diseases, mental illnesses, and substance use disorders of people living in poverty in the United States. The report concluded that recent policies seemed to be "deliberately designed to remove basic protections from the poorest, punish those who are not in employment, and make even basic health care into a privilege to be earned rather than a right of citizenship" (p. 4). In the United States, the combination of social norms (e.g., the belief that poor people are "wasters, losers, and scammers") and public policies (e.g., laws that place unattainable conditions on social welfare programs to prevent poor people from *cheating the system*, despite extremely low rates of documented welfare fraud) serves to subjugate a large number of citizens at the hands of a small minority of oppressors (Alston 2018, p. 6).

Case Study: Applying the Social Determinants of Mental Health Framework to People With Disabilities

People with disabilities are commonly overlooked (or discriminated against) in society, especially in regard to issues involving social determinants of mental health and social justice. According to recent estimates, 61 million Americans, or 25% of the population, have disabilities (Okoro et al. 2018). Despite these large numbers, people with disabilities are a highly oppressed group in U.S. society (i.e., they are often marginalized and at times are powerless). Marginalization of people with disabilities is pervasive, and they are often physically and socially othered and cordoned off from other members of society. Disabilities impact people throughout the life span, and the relative invisibility of people with disabilities (a product of this marginalization) leads to exclusion from consideration of societal advantages. In thinking about disabilities using a social determinants of mental health framework, it is apparent that young people with disabilities have worse mental health outcomes than young people without disabilities

(Honey et al. 2011). Also, because there is an indirect association between disabilities and higher rates of depression in adults, depression is classified as a secondary condition in people with disabilities (Kemp 2006). Therefore, poor mental health outcomes, and more specifically mental health inequities, exist among this population group.

Starting at the foundation of the framework (see Figure 2–1 earlier in this chapter), we might consider the social norms and public policies that set the stage for mental health inequities and poor outcomes in people with disabilities. Traditionally and historically, the United States viewed people with disabilities through the lens of the *medical model*. Prevailing social norms at the beginning of the twentieth century promoted the central idea that people with disabilities were deficient or inferior in some way. Social norms emphasized that people with disabilities were diseased or infirm, dependent on others, lacking in productivity, and unable to contribute to society in significant ways (DeJong 1994). This medical focus often emphasized impairment and deficits instead of strengths, which further led to societal beliefs that people with disabilities were lacking or inferior to others.

Naturally, public policies reflected these negative social norms about people with disabilities. Policies in the early twentieth century focused on exclusion and segregation of people with disabilities, leading to their institutionalization and relegation to asylums. The 1927 U.S. Supreme Court ruling *Buck v. Bell* upheld forced involuntary sterilization of disabled women, a precedent that endured for many years (Burgdorf and Burgdorf 1976). Other de facto policies that harmed people with disabilities have slowly begun to be addressed and reversed by federal laws. For example, the Education for All Handicapped Children Act of 1975 (renamed the Individuals with Disabilities Education Act in 1990) was the first federal policy to guarantee free and appropriate education for people with disabilities. More recently, the Americans with Disabilities Act of 1990 (which was amended in 2008) was passed to eliminate discrimination and marginalization experienced by people with disabilities. However, structural discrimination built into the creation and implementation of these laws has led to widening inequities among people of color and poor people with disabilities when compared with more affluent white people with disabilities (Beratan 2006). These attempts at progress have significant limitations and often have not gone far enough to reverse or prevent ongoing oppression that people with disabilities face in the United States (Drimmer 1992; McKenzie and Green 2019).

These social norms and public policies have also interacted with each other to create social injustice. If social norms dictate that people with disabilities are not capable of contributing productively to society, it follows that unwritten, informal discriminatory policies systematically exclude people with disabilities from the educational system and the workforce, increasing the likelihood that people with disabilities live with poverty, discrimination, marginalization, social isolation, and exclusion. This, in turn, has led to a host of social determinants of mental health. People with disabilities are less likely to have high school and college diplomas than are people without disabilities (U.S. Bureau of Labor Statistics 2015). In 2019, the unemployment rate for people with disabilities (7.3%) was double the unemployment rate for people without disabilities (3.4%) (U.S. Bureau of Labor Statistics 2020). Compared with people who do not have disabilities, people with disabilities are more likely to forgo medical care because of cost and are less likely to have household incomes greater than $15,000 or to have adequate transportation (Krahn et al. 2015).

Ultimately, as shown at the top of Figure 2–1, these social determinants of mental health lead to physiological and psychological stress, behavioral risk factors, and reduced options (often misinterpreted as poor choices) for people with disabilities, including increased obesity, increased smoking, and increased risk of being victims of violence compared with people without disabilities (Krahn et al. 2015). These are the mechanisms that lead to poor mental health outcomes and mental health inequities for people with disabilities. Critically, intervention attempts to address mental well-being must focus on changing the public policies and social norms that drive oppression and injustice that people with disabilities experience.

Taking Action to Address Social Determinants of Mental Health

Fortunately, there is a glimmer of hope. Progress is being made. In recent years, there has been an increased emphasis on the importance of screening and assessing for social determinants of health and mental health (Thomas-Henkel and Schulman 2017). Health systems in the United States have invested $2.5 billion to address the social determinants of health (Horwitz et al. 2020). Health outcomes and cost-effectiveness of such programs as they relate to housing support, nutritional support, income support, care coordination, and community outreach are being studied (Taylor et al. 2016).

Unfortunately, this progress has not resulted in closing the gap in relation to health and mental health inequities in the United States (Shim and Compton 2017). Absent from this increased focus on the social determinants of health is an understanding of the role of injustice in driving these determinants. Investments in addressing the social determinants of mental health will have minimal impact without attempting to change the public policies, social norms, and injustices that create these determinants in the first place. Without a true understanding of the forces of oppression and structural violence that are codified in our laws and policies and that lead to inequities in health, well-meaning mental health professionals may lack the moral imperative to act.

To begin to take action to address the social determinants of mental health, one must consider directly changing public policies and social norms. Many mental health professionals feel that they lack appropriate training to consider how oppression and social injustice drive social determinants of mental health. In many respects, this fear is based in some element of truth. Few mental health professionals have extensive scholarly backgrounds in oppression and social justice, in which fields such as anthropology, sociology, Black studies, queer studies, feminist studies, critical race theory, disability studies, Jewish studies, Chicano studies, Asian American studies, Indigenous studies, and many other academic disciplines have been immersed for decades. Education and self-study are important tools to increase motivation to act (see Chapter 15, "Social Justice and Advocacy," and Chapter 16, "Social Justice and Mental Health"). However, mental health professionals already possess one of the most important tools necessary to begin to bring about significant change: increased awareness. To work to correct the imbalance of advantages that have gone to wealthy, privileged communities versus the disadvantages and harm that have been directed toward oppressed and othered communities, mental health professionals should consider delivering mental health services in ways that serve to intentionally and specifically benefit those groups most disadvantaged and oppressed in society. This *preferential option for the poor* is rooted in the teachings of liberation theology and aims to reverse the damage of structural violence and social injustice (Gutiérrez 1988). It requires mental health professionals to do the difficult work of going *above and beyond* for those people who are the most exploited, marginalized, and powerless.

Currently, we as mental health professionals tend to operate with a preferential option for the privileged. We strive to provide quality care for everyone but often go the extra mile for someone who positively enacts our countertransference. Perhaps that patient reminds us of a close loved one, a dear family member, or a friend. Because most mental health professionals (especially psychiatrists) have succeeded in achieving their status from positions of privilege, the people most likely to trigger positive countertransference tend to be those who are also advantaged and privileged in society.

Furthermore, because more than half of all psychiatrists in the United States do not accept insurance in their private practices—and only 43% of psychiatric private practices accept Medicaid, in contrast to 73% of other physician specialties' private practices (Bishop et al. 2014)—many psychiatrists have limited interactions with people with serious mental illnesses or with individuals under a certain income bracket. To consider a preferential option for the poor, psychiatrists and other mental health professionals should give precedence to working in public mental health settings or to expanding their private practices to serve a more diverse patient base. This is not an easy commitment to make. Existing public policies do not prioritize these values because lower reimbursement rates, lower salaries, and understaffing make it difficult to practice outside 15-minute medication checks in public mental health settings, as well as to make reasonable margins in private practice settings. However, mental health professionals must be intentional and deliberate about redistributing their power and privilege to those who need it most.

Similarly, effective interventions are not designed with a preferential option for the poor in mind. For example, some mental health professionals balk at completing disability paperwork to help people with serious and persistent mental illnesses gain Social Security disability benefits, despite high rates of mental health disabilities within the populations they serve. Fulfilling a preferential option for the poor would prioritize these activities as an important part of ensuring the mental well-being and stability of patients. Furthermore, mental health professionals can preferentially consider the poor by approaching assessments and evaluations with a greater understanding of the structural forces that lead to poor mental health outcomes and by implementing strategies to mitigate these structural forces in the lives of their patients.

To effectively take action at a systemic level, mental health professionals, working in conjunction with various cross-sector agencies, need to influence and endorse public policies that promote mental health and well-being, which require action beyond the walls of the clinic and in partnership with policy makers. In this way, mental health professionals can use their privilege, power, and influence to connect with local, state, and federal representatives, who respond very positively to constituents who offer their expertise and assistance (Satcher and Shim 2015).

Because one role of mental health professionals is to observe, understand, comment on, and help to change social norms, we as practitioners have an important responsibility to identify, name, and speak out against social norms pertaining to social injustices such as oppression, racism, sexism, ableism, and other forms of social exclusion (Shim and Compton 2020). We must denounce those social norms that promote (or condone) exclusionary thoughts or actions, even (and especially) within the mental health profession and the broader field of medicine.

Conclusion

It was well over a decade ago that *Closing the Gap in a Generation* (Commission on Social Determinants of Health 2008) was released, and the urgency of the message is one of its most salient and enduring features. The report lamented that society had not yet prioritized fixing the avoidable conditions that lead to massive mortality gaps. "Social injustice is killing people on a grand scale," the report noted (p. 26). Faced with this realization, the lack of urgency is indeed concerning. And although the report has led to an explosion of papers, policy briefs, resolutions, and citations and spawned significant progress in the recommendation to measure, evaluate, and raise awareness about the social determinants of health, little policy action has been taken to tackle the inequitable distribution of power, money, and resources or to improve the conditions of daily life (Rasanathan 2018). If anything, the distribution of power, money, and resources in the United States has become even more unequal, and conditions of daily life have worsened. These poor living conditions and the inequitable distribution of power and resources have been laid bare during the coronavirus disease 2019 (COVID-19) pandemic (Wang and Tang 2020).

Addressing the social determinants of mental health is a moral imperative that has not been fully realized. Society's inability to make lasting positive change in this area partially stems from a failure to consider the *actual* drivers of the social determinants of mental health. When society is ready to genuinely address the social injustices that create the unfair and unjust distribution of opportunities, both in the United States and worldwide, progress may truly begin.

Questions for Self-Reflection

1. What are my associations (implicit and explicit) about people who are poor? How might this impact how I interact with them? How might this affect where I choose to practice?
2. Which patients am I most likely to go above and beyond for? What are some of the characteristics of the patients with whom I most identify?
3. What are my associations (implicit and explicit) about people with disabilities? How intentional have I been about making my services accessible to people with disabilities?

References

Alston P: Report of the Special Rapporteur on Extreme Poverty and Human Rights on His Mission to the United States of America. New York, United Nations General Assembly Human Rights Council, May 2018

Arno PS, House JS, Viola D, Schechter C: Social Security and mortality: the role of income support policies and population health in the United States. J Public Health Policy 32:234–250, 2011

Astbury J: Gender disparities in mental health, in Mental Health: A Call for Action. Edited by World Health Ministers. Geneva, Switzerland, Ministeral Round Tables 2001, 54th World Health Assembly, 2001

Baicker K, Taubman SL, Allen HL, et al: The Oregon experiment—effects of Medicaid on clinical outcomes. N Engl J Med 368:1713–1722, 2013

Barnert ES, Dudovitz R, Nelson BB, et al: How does incarcerating young people affect their adult health outcomes? Pediatrics 139:e20162624, 2017

Beitchman JH, Wilson B, Douglas L, et al: Substance use disorders in young adults with and without LD: predictive and concurrent relationships. J Learn Disabil 34:317–332, 2001

Beratan GD: Institutionalizing inequity: ableism, racism, and IDEA 2004. Disabil Stud Q 26:2, 2006

Beyer K, Kaltenbach A, Szabo A, et al: Exposure to neighborhood green space and mental health: evidence from the Survey of the Health of Wisconsin. Int J Environ Res Public Health 11:3453–3472, 2014

Bishop TF, Press MJ, Keyhani S, Pincus HA: Acceptance of insurance by psychiatrists and the implications for access to mental health care. JAMA Psychiatry 71:176–181, 2014

Braveman P: Health difference, disparity, inequality, or inequity—What difference does it make what we call it?, in Understanding Health Inequalities and Justice: New Conversations Across the Disciplines. Edited by Buchbinder M, Rivkin-Fish M, Walker RL. Chapel Hill, University of North Carolina Press, 2016, pp 33–63

Burgdorf RL Jr, Burgdorf MP: The Wicked Witch is almost dead: Buck v. Bell and the sterilization of handicapped persons. Temple Law Q 50:995–1034, 1976

Burns JK, Tomita A, Kapadia AS: Income inequality and schizophrenia: increased schizophrenia incidence in countries with high levels of income inequality. Int J Soc Psychiatry 60:185–196, 2014

Chartier K, Caetano R: Ethnicity and health disparities in alcohol research. Alcohol Res Health 33:152–160, 2010

Clark C, Ryan L, Kawachi I, et al: Witnessing community violence in residential neighborhoods: a mental health hazard for urban women. J Urban Health 85:22–38, 2008

Clements-Nolle K, Marx R, Katz M: Attempted suicide among transgender persons: the influence of gender-based discrimination and victimization. J Homosex 51:53–69, 2006

Commission on Social Determinants of Health: Closing the Gap in a Generation: Health Equity Through Action on the Social Determinants of Health. Final Report of the Commission on Social Determinants of Health. Geneva, Switzerland, World Health Organization, 2008

Compton MT, Shim RS (eds): The Social Determinants of Mental Health. Arlington, VA, American Psychiatric Publishing, 2015

Compton WM, Gfroerer J, Conway KP, Finger MS: Unemployment and substance outcomes in the United States 2002–2010. Drug Alcohol Depend 142:350–353, 2014

Davey-Rothwell MA, German D, Latkin CA: Residential transience and depression: does the relationship exist for men and women? J Urban Health 85:707–716, 2008

DeJong G: Toward a research and training capacity in disability policy. Policy Stud J 22:152–160, 1994

DeWitt L: The decision to exclude agricultural and domestic workers from the 1935 Social Security Act. Soc Secur Bull 70:49, 2010

Drimmer JC: Cripples, overcomers, and civil rights: tracing the evolution of federal legislation and social policy for people with disabilities. UCLA Law Rev 40:1341–1410, 1992

Farmer PE, Nizeye B, Stulac S, Keshavjee S: Structural violence and clinical medicine. PLoS Med 3:e449, 2006

Freire P: Pedagogy of the Oppressed, 30th Anniversary Edition. New York, Continuum International Publishing Group, 1970

Galtung J: Violence, peace, and peace research. J Peace Res 6:167–91, 1969

Green KE, Feinstein BA: Substance use in lesbian, gay, and bisexual populations: an update on empirical research and implications for treatment. Psychol Addict Behav 26:265–278, 2012

Gutiérrez G: A Theology of Liberation: History, Politics, and Salvation. New York, Orbis, 1988

Hjorth CF, Bilgrav L, Frandsen LS, et al: Mental health and school dropout across educational levels and genders: a 4.8-year follow-up study. BMC Public Health 16:976, 2016

Horwitz LI, Chang C, Arcilla HN, Knickman JR: Quantifying health systems' investment in social determinants of health, by sector, 2017–19. Health Aff (Millwood) 39(2):192–198, 2020

Honey A, Emerson E, Llewellyn G: The mental health of young people with disabilities: impact of social conditions. Soc Psychiatry Psychiatr Epidemiol 46:1–10, 2011

Iritani BJ, Bonita J, Hallfors DD, Bauer DJ: Crystal methamphetamine use among young adults in the USA. Addiction 102:1102–1113, 2007

Kemp B: Depression as a secondary condition in people with disablties, in Workshop on Disability in America: A New Look-Summary and Background Papers. Washington, DC, Institute of Medicine, 2006, pp. 234–250

Krahn GL, Walker DK, Correa-De-Araujo R: Persons with disabilities as an unrecognized health disparity population. Am J Public Health 105:S198–S206, 2015

Martin E: The egg and the sperm: how science has constructed a romance based on stereotypical male-female roles. Signs 16:485–501, 1991

McKenzie JM, Green AL: The Individuals with Disabilities Education Act: the further marginalization of racially and ethnically diverse students for more than 40 years, in The Complex Web of Inequality in North American Schools. Edited by Conchas GQ, Hinga BM, Abad MN, Gutiérrez KD. New York, Routledge, 2019, pp 173–168

Melis G, Gelormino E, Marra G, et al: The effects of the urban built environment on mental health: a cohort study in a large northern Italian city. Int J Envrion Res Public Health 12:14898–14915, 2015

Merrick MT, Ports KA, Ford DC, et al: Unpacking the impact of adverse childhood experiences on adult mental health. Child Abuse Negl 69:10–19, 2017

Nikulina V, Widom CS, Czaja S: The role of childhood neglect and childhood poverty in predicting mental health, academic achievement and crime in adulthood. Am J Community Psychol 48:309–321, 2011

Okoro CA, Hollis ND, Cyrus AC, Griffin-Blake S: Prevalence of disabilities and health care access by disability status and type among adults: United States, 2016. MMWR Morb Mortal Wkly Rep 67:882–887, 2018

Paradies Y, Ben J, Denson N, et al: Racism as a determinant of health: a systematic review and meta-analysis. PLoS One 10:e0138511, 2015

Parks J, Svendsen D, Singer P, et al: Morbidity and Mortality in People with Serious Mental Illness. Alexandria, VA, National Association of State Mental Health Program Directors Medical Directors Council, 2006

Parrott S, Aron-Dine A, Rosenbaum D et al: Trump budget deeply cuts health, housing, other assistance for low-and moderate-income families. Washington, DC, Center on Budget and Policy Priorities, February 14, 2018. Available at: www.cbpp.org/sites/default/files/atoms/files/2-14-18bud.pdf. Accessed May 4, 2020.

Pryor L, Lioret S, Van Der Waerden J, et al: Food insecurity and mental health problems among a community sample of young adults. Soc Psychiatry Psychiatr Epidemiol 51:1073–1081, 2016

Rasanathan K: 10 Years after the Commission on Social Determinants of Health: social injustice is still killing on a grand scale. Lancet 392:1176–1177, 2018

Roberts S, Arseneault L, Barratt B, et al: Exploration of NO2 and PM2.5 air pollution and mental health problems using high-resolution data in London-based children from a UK longitudinal cohort study. Psychiatry Res 272:8–17, 2019

Rataj E, Kunzweiler K, Garthus-Niegel S: Extreme weather events in developing countries and related injuries and mental health disorders—a systematic review. BMC Public Health 16:1020–1032, 2016

Satcher D, Shim RS: A call to action: addressing the social determinants of mental health, in The Social Determinants of Mental Health, Compton MT, Shim RS, Eds. Arlington, VA, American Psychiatric Publishing, 2015, pp 77–98

Shim RS, Compton MT: Measuring up on mental health? Lessons learned from the Healthy People 2020 Midcourse Review. Psychiatr Times 34(12), December 21, 2017

Shim RS, Compton MT: The social determinants of mental health, in The American Psychiatric Association Publishing Textbook of Psychiatry, 7th Edition. Edited by Roberts LW. Washington, DC, American Psychiatric Publishing, 2019, pp 163–176

Shim RS, Compton MT: The social determinants of mental health: psychiatrists' roles in addressing discrimination and food insecurity. FOCUS 18:25–30, 2020

Silver E, Mulvey EP, Swanson JW: Neighborhood structural characteristics and mental disorder: Faris and Dunham revisited. Soc Sci Med 55:1457–1470, 2002

Taylor LA, Tan AX, Coyle CE, et al: Leveraging the social determinants of health: what works? PLoS One 11(8):e0160217, 2016

Thomas-Henkel C, Schulman M: Screening for social determinants of health in populations with complex needs: implementation and considerations. Hamilton, NJ, Center for Health Care Strategies, October 2017. Available at: www.chcs.org/media/SDOH-Complex-Care-Screening-Brief-102617.pdf. Accessed September 5, 2020.

U.S. Bureau of Labor Statistics: People with a disability less likely to have completed a bachelor's degree. TED: The Economics Daily, July 20, 2015. Available at: www.bls.gov/opub/ted/2015/people-with-a-disability-less-likely-to-have-completed-a-bachelors-degree.htm. Accessed May 8, 2020.

U.S. Bureau of Labor Statistics: Persons with a disability: labor force characteristics summary. Economic News Release, February 26, 2020. Available at: www.bls.gov/news.release/disabl.nr0.htm. Accessed May 8, 2020.

U.S. Department of Health and Human Services: Mental Health: Culture, Race, and Ethnicity—A Supplement to Mental Health: A Report of the Surgeon General. Rockville, MD, Substance Abuse and Mental Health Services Administration, 2001

Wang Z, Tang K: Combating COVID-19: health equity matters. Nat Med 26:458–458, 2020

Wolff EN: The distribution of household wealth: methodological issues, time trends, and cross-sectional comparisons, in Economic Inequality and Poverty: International Perspectives. Philadelphia, PA, Taylor and Francis, 2017, pp. 92–133

World Health Organization: Social determinants of health. Geneva, Switzerland, World Health Organization, 2020. Available at: www.who.int/social_determinants/sdh_definition/en. Accessed April 29, 2020.

CHAPTER 3

Social Injustice and Mental Health Inequities

Sonya M. Shadravan, M.D.
Nicolás E. Barceló, M.D.

[D]ata never speak for themselves. It is the questions we pose (and those we fail to ask) as well as our theories, concepts, and ideas that bring a narrative and meaning to marginal distributions, correlations, regression coefficients, and statistics of all kinds.

Lawrence D. Bobo

The World Health Organization (2020) defines *health inequalities* as differences in health or determinants of health between various population groups. Some of the determinants of these differences in outcomes or health status may be the result of unavoidable factors, such as the process of aging. In contrast, when uneven distributions or outcomes may be avoidable and unjust, these are referred to as *health inequities* (World Health Organization 2020).

When examining disparities, or differing distributions of outcomes, in mental health (Krieger 1999), the tendency within public health and medical discourse is to reflexively think about the *what* of the problem. The following are examples of such thinking:

- "What are the rates of conduct disorders in Black youth compared with white youth?"
- "What are the best evidence-based treatments for women diagnosed with borderline personality disorder?"
- "What is the prevalence of suicide attempts among sexual minority and gender-nonconforming youth?"

Researchers collect data, create logistical regression models, and publish these differences, hoping that the data will speak for themselves. Although these inquiries and efforts are usually well meaning, they do not get at the heart of the processes that have created and continue to create and perpetuate unnecessary, avoidable, unjust, and unfair systems and health outcomes (Krieger 1994).

Therefore, in grappling with understanding inequity and its function and persistence through time, we propose in this chapter a focus on process over content—on the *hows* of inequity rather than the *whats*. By emphasizing the importance of nuance in terminology and theoretical frameworks, we explore how current frames of thought have come to be and how difference has been and continues to be manufactured under scientific and health frameworks. Additionally, we examine how sociohistorical context is often erased from health frameworks and how this impairs the ability to understand mental health inequities. We explore how inequity is perpetuated not only through what is studied, named, and seen but also by what is made invisible and whose positionality is left unnamed and unquestioned.

On Process, Precision, and Theory

Most often, the catalysts of inequity are not only specific policies but also processes that are blindly perpetuated, concepts that are taken for granted, and variables that go unspecified. In mental health, one often sees cavalier interchanging of terms such as *culture*, *race*, *ethnicity*, and *diversity* or *sex* and *gender*, for example. This kind of imprecision in language and theory allows inequity to be misnamed, misidentified, and thereby perpetuated (Krieger et al. 2010). Health professionals must elevate the precision of discourse on mental health inequities. This requires promoting intellectual humility by turning to our colleagues in the social sciences, who have many decades of experience in exploring these topics, to strengthen our understanding through the use of clear and precise working definitions and theoretical frameworks.

Vectors of Inequity: Shapeshifting Through Time and Space

Vectors, commonly thought of as transmitters of disease, can also be useful metaphors for understanding the subtle ways in which inequity is propagated. In keeping with a focus on the *hows* and processes, it is crucial to recognize that the systems that create and perpetuate inequities transmute and shapeshift through time, while the underlying motivating forces and impacts remain intact (Ford and Airhihenbuwa 2010). For example, Michelle Alexander (2010), in her book *The New Jim Crow: Mass Incarceration in the Age of Colorblindness*, examines how the U.S. carceral system (known to many as the criminal justice system) currently facilitates widespread racial discrimination, segregation, and exclusion in a manner very similar to what was achieved during the Jim Crow era. If we fail to recognize this dynamic disguise, how vectors of inequity shapeshift, we could be convinced that the election of President Barack Obama represented the end of systemic racism in the United States or that the representative proportion of female medical students and residents is testament to the lack of sexism in medicine. If, however, we are prepared for the transmutation of injustice, we are better able to identify contemporary drivers of injustice, recognizing, as author and activist James Baldwin describes, that "there is no moral distance" between the forms of inequity from our past and those that persist today (Moore 1963).

On Essentialism and Essentializing Difference

Essentialism represents the belief that there are distinct, unchanging, and natural characteristics that define social groups and facilitate their categorization (Haslam et al. 2000). This often-unquestioned belief that things—and particularly social identities (e.g., races, ethnic groups, sexes, sexualities)—have distinct intrinsic characteristics has underscored and continues to underscore fallacies in our understanding of inequity, thereby perpetuating it. It is important to grasp some of the different ways in which essentialist thinking has rooted itself in our paradigms of thought about identity, illness, and health.

Biological Determinism

The field of medicine, since its inception, has been entrenched in pseudo-scientific and essentialist notions about biological difference and, importantly, about *hierarchies* among these manufactured and scientifically sanctioned categories. In the early 1700s, in a social context of global incentives to condone imperialism and slavery, ecologist and taxonomist Carl Linnaeus published *Systema Naturae*, in which he described four distinct racial categories: *Homo americanus* ("reddish, choleric, obstinate, contented, and regulated by custom"), *Homo europaeus* ("white..., blue-eyed, gentle, and governed by laws"), *Homo asiaticus* ("sallow..., avaricious, and ruled by opinions"), and *Homo afer* ("black, phlegmatic, cunning, lazy, lustful, careless, and governed by caprice") (Leary 2005, p. 43). Similarly, numerous researchers and physicians propagated biological determinism in medical literature, asserting, for example, that "blacks were so different from whites—less intelligent, much less sensitive to pain, possessing numerous physical anomalies as well as markedly different patterns of disease immunity—as to constitute a separate species" (Washington 2008, p. 74). Although today this literature is called *pseudoscience*, these published categories and descriptions at the time were taken as unquestioned science, and some of these beliefs have persisted in modern medical thought (Hoffman et al. 2016).

This medical fiction about biological (and moral) difference was used to justify systematic oppression and inequity both in ideology and in the practice and structures that followed suit. If *Homo americanus*, after all, were inherently "obstinate," perhaps Indigenous people's resistance to marginalization and enclosure could be more easily dismissed as an inherent trait of the race rather than a natural and normal response to state-sanctioned violence and genocide. If *Homo afer* were intrinsically "cunning, lazy, and governed by caprice or impulsivity" and possessed an inability to feel pain, it could follow in the collective conscience of those in power that enslavement and brutality were consistent with this scientific and presumed natural order. Also, if *Homo europaeus* were conveniently defined as being innately "gentle" and "lawful," oppressive regimes led by white supremacists could remain unquestioned.

These frameworks inevitably informed scientific thinking about health. For example, when J. Marion Sims, a gynecologist who experimented on enslaved Black women without anesthesia, noted increased rates of newborn tetanus in enslaved children, he attributed this to the inherent inferiority of Black women. He asserted, "Whenever there are poverty, and filth, and laziness, or where the intellectual capacity is cramped, the moral and social feelings blunted, there it will be oftener found" (Washington 2008, p. 62). In this way, the system of slavery and its role in fueling poor health is absolved, and inequity is explained as being the direct result of intrinsic attributes of oppressed people themselves.

Beyond the construction of race under the guise of science, this kind of essentialized difference among social categories has occurred when it comes to overstating or incorrectly attributing differences in sex, gender, and sexuality to inherent biological difference alone. Psychologist Linda Gannon (1998) described the way in which patriarchy relies on the othering of women through emphasis on observable or biological differences. Gannon detailed how the scientific community has overstated the role of hormones in a wide array of domains, such as by explaining women's "inferior" or "pathological" mood, performance, and behavior, despite data to the contrary. Studies purporting to examine the impact of menopausal hormone changes on women's mental health, for example, often do not measure hormonal levels directly but rather imprecisely presume their levels, thereby confounding variables and muddying outcomes (Gannon 1998). In the nineteenth century, medical assertions that women were "built around their womb" legitimized recommendations to exclude women from school and work; these sexist practices were "justified" by medical facts that women's brains, inherently different from men's brains, were wired according to particular interests, cognitive abilities, and innate patterns of behavior (Jordan-Young 2010).

In her book *Brain Storm: The Flaws in the Science of Sex Differences*, Rebecca Jordan-Young (2010) outlined the prevalence of essentialist ideas of sexuality in scientific research. She described how vast and varied beliefs about gendered sexuality have been across time and space. Despite these changing (albeit essentializing) medical narratives and social presumptions about gendered sexuality, brain organization research remains conceptually structured by "ideas about the timeless differences in the fundamental sexual natures of men and women" (Jordan-Young 2010, p. 110). These essentialized notions of gendered sexuality buttress patriarchal norms, subtly justifying the subordination of women within medical and mental health frameworks. In turn, these frameworks, thought to be objective science, inadvertently serve as vectors of inequity.

Although these examples of biological determinism in medicine's history may seem outdated, we must remember James Baldwin's assertion that "there is no moral distance" between the creation of those assertions and persistent pseudoscientific paradigms that justify inequity under the guise of objective science. In a 2016 study investigating patterns of racial bias in the assessment and treatment of pain in patients of various races, approximately 50% of white residents and medical students held false beliefs about biological differences between Black and white patients—for example, believing that "blacks' nerve endings are less sensitive than whites'" or "blacks' skin is thicker than whites'" (Hoffman et al. 2016). Holding these false beliefs about biological differences by race predicted the underassessment and undertreatment of pain in Black patients. These findings are particularly pertinent in the context of systematic undertreatment of pain in Black patients in various clinical settings (Hoffman et al. 2016). Perhaps without ever having heard of the medical assertions of the 1800s, medical students and trainees today might believe these early fallacies about essentialized difference, even without explicit instruction. Furthermore, alleged genetic explanations of racial difference perpetuate the false notion that race itself, marked by distinct and unchanging group characteristics, explains health inequities. Therefore, these beliefs distract attention from how *racism*, and not *race*, is the true determinant of health inequities at every level (Krieger et al. 2010).

Much like the politics of essentialism that fuel racial inequity, an asymmetric focus on pathologizing women and "managing" women's hormones while excluding men from similar treatment fuels gender inequity, both past and present. These patterns, therefore, require us to remember that the *what* of inequity is usually less pertinent than the *how*—that the vectors of inequity shapeshift throughout time and space and continue to inform our diagnostic tools, treatment systems, research frameworks, and even our initiatives to promote health equity.

Cultural Determinism and "Culture Talk"

In understanding that racial categories are not biologically distinct but rather are the product of social categorization in our field, the medical community has embraced the notion of *cultural competency*, and its tenets are currently employed in approximately 90% of medical school curricula (Benjamin 2017). *Culture* is commonly understood as a set of values, practices, beliefs, and meanings that are shared by a given group (Ton and Lim 2015). The cultural competency framework recognized a need for a largely racially homogeneous workforce of privileged physicians to adequately serve a "diverse" (usually intended to mean nonwhite) patient population. Although well-intentioned *in principle*, in many cases, the cultural competency model *in practice* has served as a toolkit of racial stereotypes that are presented as scientifically based, medically relevant information for doctors to increase their knowledge and self-efficacy in treating diverse populations. The following are some examples of traditional culturally competent take-home messages:

- "Chinese parents may engage in cupping—this is not always child abuse."
- "Latinas manifest anxiety in somatic ways."
- "Black people don't trust the medical system."

Cultural syndromes, as described in DSM-5 (American Psychiatric Association 2013), have the unintended consequence of pathologizing nonwhite people on the basis of the assumption of static group practices and ways of being. Culture as an idiom became the new, shapeshifted way to essentialize and manufacture differences by groups, allowing racial stereotypes and fabrications to be replaced by cultural ones (Benjamin 2017). Sociologist Ruha Benjamin (2017) underscored the propensity of the medical field to engage in "culture talk"—a way of discussing differences that flattens the complexity of social groups, ignores the context in which inequity persists, and hides the positionality (i.e., the Eurocentric vantage point) of those who perpetuate these cultural generalizations.

Thus, cultural explanations of inequities in outcomes or treatment become a more socially acceptable way of invoking the same genetic and cultural traits that were used to hierarchize groups in biological determinism, thus still fueling systematic racism and inequity. The vector shapeshifts, but the function in preserving inequity remains the same. For as long as we believe in distinct, stagnant, and innate traits of different groups, we turn to the groups themselves to explain differences in outcomes rather than acknowledging the role of systems of oppression, subjugation, and subordination that create these unjust and avoidable differences in social experience. If we truly internalize the understanding that humans do not have any intrinsically differing or hierarchized traits by group, then when we see differences in outcomes, we will begin to comprehend that oppressive forces that have differentially treated these groups are the cause of such differences.

Benjamin (2017) noted that in contrast to grappling with systemic oppression, part of the reason *culture talk* is so prevalent is that it provides "an elaborate alibi, or a proof of innocence, letting institutionalized racism and structural inequality off the hook" (p. 228). The propagation of systems (including ways of thinking, such as culture talk) that perpetuate inequities in mental health does not require malicious intent. Therefore, we cannot allow defensiveness around our good intentions to blind us from recognizing the *impact* of our practices, our language, and our frames of understanding.

Myopia and the Erasure of Context

Biological determinism and cultural determinism are prevalent practices in medical discourse that serve to distract from oppression and to explain away health inequities as inherent by-products of innate and intrinsic group differences. These practices go hand in hand with a process of erasing sociohistorical context when seeking to understand the etiology of inequity. This essentializing and erasure contributes to scientific imprecision and stunting of our understanding. Krieger et al. (2010) described how this practice of "de-politicizing and de-historicizing health inequities" (p. 749) is built into the biomedical model. At its core, the biomedical model emphasizes biological determinants of disease, the notion that populations are the sum of individuals and that broader health patterns are the product of individuals' health patterns (Krieger 1994). For example, social determinants research and literature are often replete with interventions to increase access to services for the *underserved*, while rarely exploring the processes that cause some people to be underserved in the first place (Scott-Samuel and Smith 2015).

In medical practice, risk factors for disease are studied and taught; however, context is often erased, and confounding variables, often whole identities, are erroneously listed as the risk itself. For example, a cited risk factor for metabolic syndrome, which psychiatrists are trained to closely monitor, is being "Hispanic—especially Hispanic women" (Mayo Clinic 2019). This statement represents the type of cavalier imprecision of language and terminology mentioned earlier. *Hispanic*, a term referencing a group of people who are Spanish speaking, is being interchanged with *Latinx*, which represents an ethnically heterogeneous group based on the continent of origin. The wording of that risk factor begs the question, "Does speaking Spanish, or being a woman who speaks Spanish, increase one's risk of metabolic syndrome?" Surely, this is not the intended meaning. But even if the medical literature were to cite being Latinx as a risk factor, the same line of questioning follows: "Is there something inherent about being of Latinx origin that directly increases the risk of developing metabolic syndrome?" How can this be possible if, as previously asserted, biological racial categories do not exist? To seek a more complete understanding, we must relinquish our myopic view of risk factors and seek out what structural and historical factors have caused disparate outcomes in a given socially constructed group.

Historical context illuminates the pitfalls of using social identities as risk factors for disease. The following example demonstrates the value of more precisely considering risk factors for metabolic syndrome: According to nutritional appraisals performed in Mexico in the 1940s, obesity was exceedingly rare, and it was deemed that the imposition of dietary recommendations from the United States would lower the nutritional status of Mexican people (Anderson et al. 1948). When the North American Free Trade Agreement (NAFTA) was signed in 1994, causing widespread dietary changes throughout Mexico, increased rates of obesity followed (Clark et al. 2012). Without this context, it is assumed that some inherent aspect of Latinx identity is the attributable risk for obesity. With this added context, however, medical providers may understand more deeply the social, political, and economic processes that affect obesity differentially in people in the United States. This knowledge may lead to further exploration of structural drivers of inequity: Who has access to healthy food and why? Who has a work schedule that permits time for exercise and why? Who is poor and why? These types of questions promote precision in medicine and understanding inequity. Clearly, being Spanish speaking is not a risk factor for metabolic syndrome. That idea is not only essentializing; it is also myopic in scope and scientifically incorrect.

On Positionality and the Invisibles

Biological determinism and cultural determinism turn the microscope on groups deemed *diverse* or *special* (e.g., transgender people, immigrants, women, people of color, transgender women of color) and perpetuate inequity by what is described and analyzed. However, inequity is propagated not only by what is described and named but equally by what goes undescribed, unquestioned, unnamed, and left invisible.

Structural Oppression Made Invisible

When making sense of mental health inequities in access to services, adherence to medications, adverse outcomes, and relative prevalence of various diagnoses, we too often become overly focused on individual- and interpersonal-level relationships, failing to address the role of structural factors. For example, the DSM-5 description of disruptive, impulse control, and conduct disorders contrasts them with other DSM-5 disorders that primarily involve emotional and behavioral regulation problems, asserting that the former disorders "are manifested in behaviors that...*bring the individual into significant conflict with societal norms or authority figures*" [emphasis added] (American Psychiatric Association 2013, p. 461). For these disorders, the problem is defined as a conflict between individuals and societal norms or authority; however, the societal norms or authority practices that enter into conflict with these children do not get questioned, and societal norms and authority figures do not risk receiving a DSM-5 diagnosis—they remain invisible and immune from critique. When a study finds, for example, that Black youth are more often diagnosed with conduct disorders than are their white counterparts, "cultural differences in expression of psychiatric illness" are proposed as a possible explanation of this finding (Delbello et al. 2001, p. 101). No mention is made of the extensive evidence that societal norms and authority figures disproportionately suspect dangerousness and deviance from children of color in as early as preschool age (Gilliam et al.

2016), echoing early Linnaean presumptions about Black *caprice* (see section "Biological Determinism" earlier in this chapter). Structural racism, policing, overestimation of age, and culpability of children of color are not subject to scrutiny or investigation; rather, they remain invisible, allowing the locus of blame to remain on the children themselves.

Similarly, mental health literature generally conveys the notion that transgender people are at increased risk of depression and posits this as a likely result of hormonal shifts or the diagnosis of gender dysphoria (Arayasirikul and Wilson 2019). This overreliance on hormonal explanations to describe transgender mental health echoes the research of Gannon (1998) and Jordan-Young (2010) on the medical overreliance on hormonal explanations for "gendered mood." Additionally, although the change in DSM-5 of the diagnosis of gender identity disorder to gender dysphoria was intended to reduce stigma, the criteria and general understanding of this disorder still attribute the patient's suffering to an inherent conflict or unfulfilled desire on the part of the marginalized patient. The context of the extensive and unique oppression, stigmatization, and marginalization that transgender people face daily and the structures that produce this oppression and these health inequities remain uninterrogated and largely absent from discrimination research (Arayasirikul and Wilson 2019). These structural variables are made invisible, and thereby unchallenged, while survivors of this oppression are labeled with a new, supposedly less stigmatizing disorder.

Even when it comes to matters thought to be straightforward in women's mental health, structural factors of patriarchy and gendered oppression are made invisible. For example, in regard to premenstrual dysphoric disorder and menopause, the swiftness with which women's emotions or emotional changes are medicalized, labeled, and intervened in stands in stark contrast to how men's anger and emotionality are perceived as normal, rational, or likely in response to valid distress. As Gannon (1998) described,

> If we were to accept women's anger as a legitimate response to economic, social, and political oppression, we would not assume that she is premenstrual every time she raises her voice. If we were to view men's aggression as a symptom of excessive testosterone, we would require hormonal monitoring of those men who control nuclear weapons. (p. 295)

An image that has gained great popularity in equity-minded spaces is illustrated in Figure 3–1. Although there is some value in demonstrating the need to move beyond a "color-blind" or "one-size-fits-all" approach to equity, this image does not explore *why* these three individuals are different heights in the first place. If this image is to represent equity for anything other than height and game-watching access, it would suggest that some people are, metaphorically speaking, inherently short (echoing biological and cultural determinism).

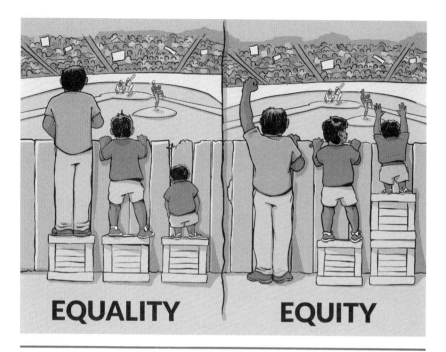

FIGURE 3–1. Depiction of the difference between equality and equity.

The image seeks to demonstrate the difference between interventions promoting equality (treating all people the same) versus equity (giving people what they need to have equal outcomes).

Source. Angus Maguire (artist), Interaction Institute for Social Change 2016. Available at: https://interactioninstitute.org/illustrating-equality-vs-equity. Accessed April 24, 2020.

To shed light on the structures and systems that make some people *appear*, for example, shorter, unhealthier, or more criminal, consider Figure 3–2. The importance of uprooting our assumptions cannot be overstated. *How* we think about difference shapes the quality of our understanding and the accountability of our interventions.

Privilege and the Positionality of Medicine Made Invisible

In addition to erasing historical context and making structural oppression invisible, macro-level forces that produce inequity (making certain groups the invisible, unnamed, normed reference point) perpetuate the marginalization of certain groups as inherently inferior or forever different. Terms and de-

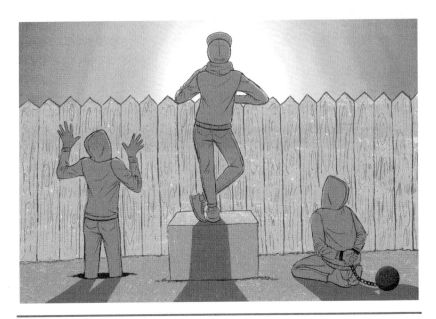

FIGURE 3–2.   Depiction of three individuals of the same true height subject to different stature-distorting conditions.

This image exposes the false assumptions about inherent inferiority or superiority that often underpin equity-based interventions.

Source.   Barcelo NE, Shadravan SM: Stop Drawing Us Short: Limitations and Possibilities in Graphic Representations of Power and Privilege. Original art by Nicolás E. Barceló, Sonya M. Shadravan, and Aria Ghalili (artist). Presented at Minority Health Conference, Los Angeles, CA, February 2020.

scriptions such as *minority mental health* or *women's mental health* or *special populations* reify the notion that mental health, or "normal" mental health, denotes white, male, insured, heterosexual, cisgender, English-speaking, able-bodied people's mental health. Many resources, toolkits, and online modules feature targeted guides for working with *diverse populations*—a term that denotes an extensive list of various communities (categorized by sex, language, ethnicity, religion, etc.)—with guides on how to work with these populations (American Psychiatric Association 2020; Centers for Disease Control and Prevention 2012; Jimenez and Lewis 2007). In addition to the problem of essentializing these imprecisely categorized groups, often what is lacking in these types of resources are any mentions of masculinity, whiteness, Christianity, or heterosexuality, for example. These attributes are left unremarked on, as the invisible norm to which all other groups are compared. Frequently, the audience is presumed to be a member of this normed white, male, heterosexual, English-speaking group, and it is presumed that only training and education on all other essentialized groups are needed.

Similarly, mental health discourse focuses on underserved populations, but communities that are *overserved* (communities with disproportionate access to resources) are never labeled as such. Mental health professionals may forget that inequity usually involves the hoarding of resources—of access, of centrality, of privilege—just as much as it involves the removal or deficit of such privilege from others. As providers are increasingly employing the biopsychosocial framework to incorporate structural understanding in their evaluations of patients' formulations and treatment plans, this pattern of invisibilizing privilege is equally made apparent. Providers list being transgender, homeless, Latinx, and uninsured as positive findings in their formulations or mental status exams while remaining taciturn on factors of privilege, such as intergenerational wealth, food security, or being white—all equally relevant in the patient's presentation and expectations, but left unmentioned, as the unquestioned norm.

In addition to reinforcing marginalization through the assumption that white, male, cisgender, financially secure individuals make up the unnamed "norm," providers have left the culture and positionality of medicine dangerously unexamined. Benjamin (2017) described the fact that the medical community labels various nonwhite groups as irrational, mistrusting of medicine, and presenting with language deficiencies, but the medical community is free of parallel scrutiny for neither gaining the trust of their patients nor providing linguistically appropriate services. For example, the American Academy of Orthopaedic Surgeons' "Cultural Tip Sheet" asserts that Asian American patients "may have an inherent distrust of Western medicine" (Jimenez and Lewis 2007). Benjamin refers to this manner of diagnosing trust issues as a *deficit approach*. Despite the supposed prevalence of distrust in so many diverse groups, providers still misattribute behaviors as fixed cultural attitudes of the individual groups themselves rather than calling into question the culture of medicine. As Benjamin (2017) suggested, "a critical race approach to the health sciences would require reorienting ourselves—away from a fixation with distrust towards the problem of institutional trustworthiness" (p. 234). From this standpoint, then, a mental health equity approach would focus less of its effort on teaching providers the fallacy that nonwhite groups are *culturally* predisposed to distrust and more toward improving trustworthiness within the mental health field.

On the Presumption of Objectivity

At the core of the aforementioned practices that fuel and disguise inequity is a presumed objectivity on the part of science and an unquestioned acceptance of research methodology, medical practice, and medical education.

The lack of humility and the presumption of fairness, despite evidence to the contrary, allow the practices of our field to perpetuate injustice while remaining off limits for critical evaluation or transformation. This presumption is what allowed the views of Linnaeus and Sims, which were direct reflections of the racist values of the times in which they lived, to be published as authoritative science (see section "Biological Determinism" earlier in this chapter). This same presumption is what allows current research on outcomes by race to list an individual's race, rather than racism, as the independent variable in measuring different outcomes. Furthermore, research methods presumed to be objective and reasonable preclude research relevant for the most marginalized populations—for example, transgender people of color or people of color with disabilities—who do not fit into the boxes neatly assigned by science. This, in turn, contributes to the erasure of certain people from our medical knowledge, as well as the suppression of any data that may challenge our predisposed expectations for population health and norms. Krieger (1999) asserted that "at issue are both acts of omission and acts of commission. These range from the virtual invisibility of lesbians and gay men in major public health databases to distortions of etiologic and therapeutic knowledge due to the underrepresentation of people of color and women in epidemiologic studies, clinical trials, and even medical textbooks" (p. 333). Public health research subscribes to traditional hierarchies of evidence (Scott-Samuel and Smith 2015) and a focus on proving causation, which typically requires a gold standard, randomized controlled trial. These valorized study designs would nonetheless be inadequate in highlighting the connection between health and structural processes. Consequently, our unwavering standards for what counts as science obfuscates the role of structural factors and subordination so essential to understanding inequity.

Conclusion

What is presented in this book are examples of the plethora of ways in which injustice is imprinted and embedded in our systems of thought, practice, and study. What we have offered in this chapter is an approach for *how* to think about the processes and paradigms that allow inequity to flourish and shapeshift through time. These processes facilitate the misnaming of problems—through imprecision in terminology; through essentializing difference; and through making invisible the role of subordination, privilege, and the subjectivity of scientific practice. These processes, in turn, beget misidentified solutions, often glorifying privileged "saviors" and devising downstream social interventions, while never questioning the determinants of the determinants or the positionality of those leading interventions to help.

Questions for Self-Reflection

1. What are the times in my professional education or continuing education when equity issues were presented as cultural ones?
2. How can I be more intentional in my acknowledgment of privilege and positionality in medicine?
3. How can I transition to focusing on the *how* and *why* of mental health inequities rather than the *what*?

References

Alexander M: The New Jim Crow: Mass Incarceration in the Age of Colorblindness. New York, The New Press, 2010

American Psychiatric Association: Diagnostic and Statistical Manual of Mental Disorders, 5th Edition. Arlington, VA, American Psychiatric Association, 2013

American Psychiatric Association: Diversity and Health Equity: Education. Washington, DC, American Psychiatric Association, 2020. Available at: www.psychiatry.org/psychiatrists/cultural-competency/education. Accessed January 1, 2020.

Anderson RK, Calvo J, Robinson W, et al: Nutritional appraisals in Mexico. Am J Public Health 38:1126–1135, 1948

Arayasirikul S, Wilson EC: Spilling the T on trans-misogyny and microaggressions: an intersectional oppression and social process among trans women. J Homosex 66:1415–1438, 2019

Benjamin R: Cultura obscura: race, power, and "culture talk" in the health sciences. Am J Law Med 43:225–238, 2017

Centers for Disease Control and Prevention: Cultural Insights: Communicating with Hispanics/Latinos. Atlanta, GA, Centers for Disease Control and Prevention, 2012. Available at: www.cdc.gov/healthcommunication/pdf/audience/audience insight_culturalinsights.pdf. Accessed January 1, 2020.

Clark SE, Hawkes C, Murphy SME, et al: Exporting obesity: U.S. farm and trade policy and the transformation of the Mexican consumer food environment. Int J Occup Environ Health 18:53–65, 2012

Delbello MP, Lopez-Larson MP, Soutullo CA, Strakowski SM: Effects of race on psychiatric diagnosis of hospitalized adolescents: a retrospective chart review. J Child Adolesc Psychopharmacol 11:95–103, 2001

Ford CL, Airhihenbuwa CO: The public health critical race methodology: praxis for antiracism research. Soc Sci Med 71:1390–1398, 2010

Gannon L: Influence of medical and sexual politics on women's health. Fem Psychol 8:285–302, 1998

Gilliam WS, Maupin AN, Reyes CR, et al: Do Early Educators' Implicit Biases Regarding Sex and Race Relate to Behavior Expectations and Recommendations of Preschool Expulsions and Suspensions? New Haven, Yale University Child Study Center, 2016

Haslam N, Rothschild L, Ernst D: Essentialist beliefs about social categories. Br J Soc Psychol 39:113–127, 2000

Hoffman KM, Trawalter S, Axt JR, Oliver MN: Racial bias in pain assessment and treatment recommendations, and false beliefs about biological differences between blacks and whites. Proc Natl Acad Sci USA 113:4296–4301, 2016

Jimenez RL, Lewis VO (eds): Culturally Competent Care Guidebook: Companion to the Cultural Competency Challenge CD-ROM. Rosemont, IL, American Academy of Orthopaedic Surgeons, 2007

Jordan-Young RM: Brain Storm: The Flaws in the Science of Sex Differences, Cambridge, MA, Harvard University Press, 2010

Krieger N: Epidemiology and the web of causation: has anyone seen the spider? Soc Sci Med 39:887–903, 1994

Krieger N: Embodying inequality: a review of concepts, measures, and methods for studying health consequences of discrimination. Int J Health Serv 29:295–352, 1999

Krieger N, Alegría M, Almeida-Filho N, et al: Who, and what, causes health inequities? Reflections on emerging debates from an exploratory Latin American/North American workshop. J Epidemiol Community Health 64:747–749, 2010

Leary J: Post Traumatic Slave Syndrome: America's Legacy of Enduring Injury and Healing. Milwaukie, MN, Uptone, 2005

Mayo Clinic: Metabolic Syndrome. Rochester, MN, Mayo Clinic, 2019. Available at: www.mayoclinic.org/diseases-conditions/metabolic-syndrome/symptoms-causes/syc-20351916. Accessed April 23, 2020.

Moore RO: Take This Hammer (documentary film). National Educational Television, 1963

Scott-Samuel A, Smith KE: Fantasy paradigms of health inequalities: utopian thinking? Soc Theory Health 13:418–436, 2015

Ton H, Lim RF: Assessment of culturally diverse individuals: introductions and formulations, in Clinical Manual of Cultural Psychiatry, 2nd Edition. Edited by Lim RF. Arlington, VA, American Psychiatric Publishing, 2015, pp 1–37

Washington H: Medical Apartheid: The Dark History of Medical Experimentation on Black Americans from Colonial Times to the Present. New York, Random House, 2008

World Health Organization: WHO Health Impact Assessment—Glossary of Terms Used. Geneva, Switzerland, 2020. Available at: www.who.int/hia/about/glos/en/index1.html. Accessed April 23, 2020.

CHAPTER 4

Social Injustice and Structural Racism

Matthew L. Edwards, M.D.
Samuel Ricardo Saenz, M.D., M.P.H.
Roy Collins, M.D., M.P.H.
Belinda Bandstra, M.D., M.A.

In this chapter, we highlight social systems and structures that create mental health disparities, cause suffering, and maintain inequities in the United States. Although such structures are known to impact the psychological well-being of people who are racially, ethnically, and experientially oppressed, we focus here on racialized systems as a case study, exploring historical narratives and current issues in structural racism and mental health. We examine these issues in hopes that mental health professionals and policy makers may better intervene to promote not only racial justice but all forms of social justice in mental health.

Researchers have frequently explored the questions of how and why mental health disparities persist. In a landmark paper titled "Social Causes as Fundamental Causes of Disease," public health scientists Link and Phelan (1995) examined the historical relationship between social life and illness, advancing a progressive framework to address the persistence of health inequities in the United States. In it, they argued that "social factors such as socioeconomic status and social support are likely 'fundamental causes' of disease" that serve to create and maintain inequity (Link and Phelan 1995, p. 80). Although this model of fundamental causes included such factors as race, income, gender, and social status, it did not fully capture the impact of racism in health inequity in that racially stigmatized groups have poorer health outcomes compared with their white counterparts, regardless of differences in socioeconomic status. Indeed, one study estimated that racial discrimination might explain as much as 15% of the variance in psychological distress and mental health symptoms among Black people, even when controlling for other contextual factors, such as age, gender, education, social class, and generic stressors (Klonoff et al. 1999). People who are racially and ethnically oppressed have higher rates of disease (often with earlier onset and increased severity of illness), are more likely to die prematurely because of disease, and are less likely to have access to medical care (U.S. Department of Health and Human Services 2001; Williams and McAdams-Mahmoud 2019). Even when racial minorities access health care, they often receive poorer quality medical care than that given to their white counterparts (Williams and McAdams-Mahmoud 2019).

Racism is also a critical psychosocial stressor. It leads to behaviors and factors (e.g., residential segregation; decreased access to resources; increased exposure to interpersonal violence, trauma, substance use, and criminal activity) associated with increased adverse health risks and poor health outcomes (Williams and McAdams-Mahmoud 2019). Moreover, the various causes of inequity are associated. For example, ostensibly race-neutral differences in the rate of criminal offenses are linked to differences in employment opportunities, discrimination, and residential segregation (Asad and Clair 2018). At the same time, people who are racially and ethnically oppressed are overrepresented in the carceral (criminal justice) system, experiencing more severe punitive consequences for behaviors such as drug offenses and misdemeanors than their white counterparts (Asad and Clair 2018; Dudley 2019). These racial differences perpetuate inequities, including in schooling, financial, and carceral systems, all of which affect health. Public discourse historically has been reluctant to link racism to poor mental health outcomes.

Definitions

What is *structural racism*? To understand structural racism, we must define both *racism* and *social structures*. Racism in the United States has roots in the Atlantic slave trade and developed to justify the social and political superiority of whites over other racial groups on the basis of physical characteristics attributed to biological differences (Fernando 2017). As such, *race* is fundamentally a socially determined, rather than biological, construct. We understand this because no single gene or cluster of genes is uniquely common to any one race. Moreover, individuals within the same population or racial group can have more genetic difference than individuals across racial groups (Witherspoon et al. 2007). In other words, an individual's race conveys more information about how he or she is perceived in society than about his or her genetic identity. Thus, there is no biological (or genetic) reason that can explain why, for example, Black Americans have poorer health outcomes in the United States than their white counterparts do.

Perceptions of race change over time within a population and differ across social contexts. An individual whose race is *Black* in the United States may be considered *white* in other racialized countries such as Brazil or the Dominican Republic (Monk 2016). Before the 1950s, Irish, Italian, Polish, Jewish, and German immigrants were primarily classified by their country of origin. As racial tensions between white and Black Americans heightened during this interwar period, these immigrant groups gradually coalesced into a white American majority (Bayor 2009). In this way, their shared physical characteristics (e.g., skin color), social behaviors (e.g., voting), and ability to acculturate into the white American majority became more important than their previously divergent national identities (Painter 2011). As this example demonstrates, racial categories in the United States can be understood only within the social and historical contexts during which they were perceived or constructed.

A race, like any social group, may be subject to prejudice and discrimination. *Prejudice* most often refers to preconceived negative beliefs or attitudes held by one group toward another that are rarely reality or evidence based (Giddens et al. 2008). Whereas prejudice describes an affect, *discrimination* refers to behaviors that create an unequal treatment or an inequitable distribution of resources based on identity or group membership (Giddens et al. 2008). Although prejudice and discrimination are different phenomena, prejudiced attitudes often lead to discriminatory practices.

Racism is defined as an "organized system premised on the categorization and ranking of social groups into races and devalues, disempowers, and differentially allocates desirable societal opportunities and resources to racial groups regarded as inferior" (Williams and Mohammed 2013, p. 2). Note that this definition goes beyond mere prejudice and discrimination practiced at an interpersonal level. A common misconception about racism is that it is a static, ideological phenomenon mostly limited to ideas and beliefs that lead individuals to commit overtly prejudicial or discriminatory practices. Although these practices certainly exist, this narrow view of racism accounts for neither the changes in racism across societies over time nor the ways in which the practices limit the opportunities and experiences of racially marginalized groups in society (Bonilla-Silva 1997). Williams and Mohammed (2013) distinguished the climate of negative stereotypes and discrimination against particular ethnic or racial groups from the policies and procedures that reduce access to social resources, such as housing, education, and employment opportunities. We consider the former *cultural* or *interpersonal racism* and the latter *structural* or *institutional racism*.

Social structures are systemic, hierarchical arrangements of economic, political, legal, religious, and cultural systems in societies. Although they are inevitable and, in some cases, necessary for the functioning of a society, social structures can stratify roles and positions such that certain groups maintain their privileged status over others. *Structural racism* engenders race-based inequity through a range of mechanisms, including residential and other forms of spatial segregation, inequitable distribution of financial resources, disproportionate criminalization, unfair employment practices, and differences in access to quality health care (Bailey et al. 2017). Unlike interpersonal prejudice and racist practices characterized by outwardly hostile, aversive, or discriminatory social behaviors, structural racism operates by normalizing social and institutional practices that reinforce socioeconomic and political differences among groups (Bonilla-Silva 1997). Moreover, historical efforts to denounce race without addressing systemic racism and implicit bias in health care settings often perpetuate racial and social inequities (see section "Racial Bias and Racialization in Mental Health Policy and Research" (Doyle 2016; Raz 2011, 2013).

Structural racism intersects with mental health in multiple ways. In this chapter, we discuss structural racism through several mechanisms, illustrating how people who are racially and ethnically oppressed can be ensconced in systems that subject them to negative social determinants of mental health over time. First of all, systems and policies may perpetuate inequities by disproportionately impacting the mental health and well-being of a particular racial or ethnic group. Second, bias and discrimination, whether explicit or implicit, by individuals and systems in positions of power within mental health can develop and preserve systems that work against racially oppressed populations at multiple levels. Mental health professionals and policy makers must understand structural racism, however subtle it may seem, to promote the mental health of people who are racially and ethnically oppressed.

Policies That Support Racialization and Race-Based Mental Health Inequities

Acculturation

For many decades, researchers and social scientists primarily focused attention on cultural differences between Latin American and U.S. cultures to explain poorer health outcomes among Latinx populations. This literature focused heavily on *acculturation*, an individual-level process through which individuals acquire the "behaviors, attitudes, and values prevalent within American society" (Lopez-Class et al. 2011, p. 1558). In this framework, culture influences the individual behaviors associated with poor health outcomes (e.g., alcohol use, smoking, dietary habits) through social norms that presumably fluctuate during the immigration process. Moreover, this literature suggests that immigrant health worsens as individuals acculturate and adopt lifestyles of the dominant American society (Escarce et al. 2006).

Although acculturation may sometimes lead to poor mental health outcomes, it does not fully explain the causes of those outcomes. Proposed interventions operating within this framework often work at the individual level. As such, they may inadvertently place the onus for improving health outcomes on individuals. Accordingly, acculturation may distract mental health professionals and policy makers from addressing the pervasive and systemic structural factors that perpetuate health inequities among immigrants. Rather than focus exclusively on individual-level characteristics and explanatory models, mental health professionals should address root structural causes contributing to the stress associated with immigration. For example, evidence suggests that punitive immigration policies, such as barring future admission for prior offenses, placement in U.S. detention centers, and deportation, explain a significant proportion of mental illness and stress, particularly in Latinx immigrant communities (Asad and Clair 2018).

Immigration Policies and Exposure to Chronic and Acute Stressors

U.S. immigration policy makers have systematically redefined legal immigration policies to legitimize racial segregation. The clearest early example of such policies is the Naturalization Act of 1790, which effectively limited pathways to citizenship to only free white people. Contemporary immigration policies echo the same racism and xenophobia that drove early U.S. anti-immigrant policies. For example, modern immigration control continues the restrictive policies first developed during periods of profound xenophobia, including quotas and exclusion of individuals who are likely to be public charges or who exhibit undesirable traits. The per-country ceiling limits immigration from any one country to 7% of the total annual immigrants to the United States (Kandel 2018). More specifically, mandatory medical examinations screen for general medical conditions, disease-specific laboratory findings, and mental disorders and substance use among foreigners applying for entry into the United States (Gee and Ford 2011). Disqualifying mental health conditions are DSM diagnoses associated with "harmful behavior" (American Psychiatric Association 2013; Centers for Disease Control and Prevention 2017). These conditions may include major depressive disorder, bipolar disorder, schizophrenia, personality disorders, anxiety disorders, sexual disorders, trauma- and stressor-related disorders, cognitive disorders, and intellectual disability, as assessed by a comprehensive psychiatric examination and psychometric instruments such as the Primary Care Evaluation of Mental Disorders (PRIME-MD), Patient Health Questionnaire–9 (PHQ-9), PTSD Checklist–Civilian version (PCL-C), and Harvard Trauma Questionnaire (HTQ) (Centers for Disease Control and Prevention 2012).

The use of medical screenings reflects a broad generalization of certain individuals seeking legal migration as inherently prone to illness or troubling behaviors, without appreciation of the disadvantageous predisposing and precipitating circumstances beyond those individuals' control. Screening documented immigrants for deleterious health conditions and characteristics leads to denial of entry for less healthy individuals, resulting in better health of immigrants on average when compared with native-born U.S. citizens and undocumented immigrants (Gee and Ford 2011). These policies lead to perceptions that individuals who immigrate from certain ethnic backgrounds have fewer health issues than those who live in the United States, which may reinforce unproven assumptions of racial or biological inferiority of Black and Latinx Americans.

These practices are associated with stress, trauma, and mental illness. Moreover, the Patient Protection and Affordable Care Act of 2010 banned undocumented immigrants from receiving health care coverage in the United States and even stipulated certain restrictions on documented immigrants. These structural restrictions serve to reinforce racial health inequities by preventing immigrants from accessing appropriate health care.

Undocumented Latinx immigrants are at an increasingly higher risk for depression, anxiety, and other mental health disorders due to stress and trauma during and after migration (Garcini et al. 2017). The high rate of mental illness in this population may be a symptom of social stressors, including the threat of deportation, financial burden, limited access to resources and opportunities that promote educational and occupational advancement, vulnerability to exploitation, and lack of social support or connections in their new country. Importantly, mental health issues among Latinx populations are particularly affected by varying state-level immigration policies. Latinx people in states with more exclusionary immigration policies report poorer mental health compared with those living in states with less exclusionary policies (Hatzenbuehler et al. 2017). *Racialized legal status* refers to legal classifications, such as immigration and criminalization status, that disproportionately affect racially and ethnically oppressed persons (Asad and Clair 2018). The consequences of racialized legal statuses also influence the perceptions, treatment, and consequently health outcomes of other members of those racial groups, regardless of their actual legal status. In other words, broader anti-immigrant climates, structured by racialized legal status, may significantly contribute to discrimination, stress, and mental illness for both immigrant and native-born populations (Asad and Clair 2018).

The threat of detention or deportation primarily targeted against Latinx immigrants (Asad and Clair 2018) and the limitations on immigrants' mobility due to fears of deportation are also associated with higher mental health needs among immigrant communities (Nichols et al. 2018). Although previous experiences with detention, deportation, or immigration officials may heighten immigrants' sense of vulnerability to future legal action, even immigrants without such experiences harbor fears of detention or deportation (Asad and Clair 2018). Removing marginalized patients facing deportation from their trusted communities is yet another challenging structural barrier to accessing appropriate mental health care. Although undocumented status negatively affects immigrants' health and well-being, gaining legal immigration status is associated with improved psychological well-being (Patler and Pirtle 2018). Policies that allow pathways to legal immigration status are examples of critical structural interventions to support the psychiatric health of immigrant populations.

Undocumented patients must navigate a precarious legal terrain. Not only do they often flee traumatic situations in their countries of origin, but because of structural racism inherent in immigration policies, they are also confronted with experiences fraught with tension and hostility in the United States. At the same time, it is vital for mental health professionals to appreciate the confluence of many intersectional, or additive, marginalized identities that contribute to these patients' experience of mental illnesses. Factors that make this population particularly vulnerable include socioeconomic needs, undocumented immigration status, foreign nationality, language barriers, and other challenges with navigating the health care system. As the country's demographic and political landscapes continue to evolve, mental health professionals may encounter patients with one or more of these challenges. They should, therefore, be prepared to address the barriers that immigrant patients face when navigating the U.S. health care system.

Racial Bias and Racialization in Mental Health Diagnosis and Screening

Racialized diagnoses and diagnostic tools make up one way in which race influences the treatment of marginalized groups. Scholars argue that "racist attitudes [are] embedded within the (psychiatric) diagnostic process" (Fernando 2017, p. 93). Assessments are conducted in a supposedly race-neutral, *objective* way, but the way psychiatry conceptualizes psychopathology is heavily influenced by historical European thought. Because of this, what is considered normative, or outside the norm, is shaped by the dominant culture. Culture bias ranges from the content and assumptions that underlie our assessments to the lack of cultural diversity of groups on which assessments are normalized (Council of National Psychological Associations for the Advancement of Ethnic Minority Interests 2016). The failure to consider how race and culture intersect class, gender, and socioeconomic issues and how these influences shape diagnostic assessment, treatment, and health outcomes is yet another example of how structural racism is built into mental health care.

Features of mental health such as "guilt, self-depreciation, depression, feelings of passivity" (Fernando 2017, p. 93) are not objective measures but rather are socially constructed concepts that reflect in part the values and assumptions of psychiatrists. Seemingly objective assessments of mental states, ranging from depressive feelings and emotional states to thought disorder and psychosis, are all assessments that grew out of psychiatric research and thought within a particular social, cultural, and institutional context. These forms of diagnostic bias may in part account for the over-representation of Black men with schizophrenia and individuals involuntarily committed to mental institutions. Although both Black and white psychiatrists have overdiagnosed schizophrenia in Black populations, studies show that white psychiatrists do so more often (Fernando 2017). This finding reflects the fact that the majority of medical educators, institutions, and research through which Black and white physicians are trained are still underrepresentative of the racial and ethnic diversity of society. Moreover, Black patients are more likely to be described as violent, dangerous, impulsive, or suspicious and more likely to have their behavior assumed to be illegal (Dudley 2019; Fernando 2017). Racial differences in paranoia and other rating scales are also observed in standardized psychometric assessments such as the Minnesota Multiphasic Personality Inventory (MMPI). There is no clinical or objective evidence to support racial differences in psychopathology and personality, and because the research on racial differences in MMPI scales remains largely equivocal, the use of the MMPI in nonwhite populations is controversial (Frueh et al. 2002; Hutton et al. 1992; McCreary and Padilla 1977). The fact that such psychometric assessments are acceptable in mental health practice without meeting more rigorous standards for validity is itself another example of structural racism.

Diagnostic racial bias exists not only in the way physicians are trained intersubjectively to assess for symptomatology but also in the diagnostic screening tools used to manage population health. Structural racism is codified in biased screening tools, diagnostic instruments, and conceptual frameworks that are not normalized for nonwhite populations (Baker and Bell 1999; Obermeyer et al. 2019). In a recent study, Obermeyer et al. (2019) reported that a widely used commercial algorithm that assesses the need for health services for more than 200 million Americans systematically favored ill white patients over Black patients, such that Black patients had significantly more symptoms of uncontrolled illness than white patients, despite similar risk estimates. As a result, Black people screened for services on the basis of risk estimates received those services at a rate of roughly one-third of what their actual health conditions would dictate, perpetuating societal biases at the population level.

Thus, although screening instruments and diagnostic aids may help standardize diagnostic procedures and criteria, these tools must be developed, tested, and validated with various target populations in mind, lest they perpetuate the biases inherent in their development (Baker and Bell 1999). Research suggests that more widely applied instruments such as the Center for Epidemiologic Studies Depression Scale (CES-D) may be more reliable when assessing individuals across different racial groups than more specialized scales such as the Geriatric Depression Scale (GDS) (Baker and Bell 1999). Moreover, there is a lack of health outcomes studies and clinical interventional studies focusing on age cohort differences, psychiatric and substance use comorbidities, and varying resource needs. The underrepresentation of Black, Latinx, Indigenous, Asian American, and multiracial groups in clinical studies and trials may contribute to the further perpetuation of biases in diagnosis and treatment (Baker and Bell 1999). More research is needed to examine the psychometric validity of commonly used mental health screening tools for groups that are racially and ethnically oppressed.

Race-based thinking can have enduring consequences for population health. These consequences include differences in diagnoses and treatment and ultimately outcomes. Studies demonstrate that even individuals who embrace egalitarian beliefs may have unconscious biases that affect patient care (Kugelmass 2016). Racial discordance between physicians and patients may trigger implicit race- and class-based assumptions that affect patient care (Kugelmass 2016). Assuming genetic differences between various races may lead to damaging clinical repercussions, including overdiagnosis and underdiagnosis of illness (Wailoo and Pemberton 2006). Even among clinicians who correct for incorrect explicit beliefs, implicit bias may still lead to an unintentional misunderstanding of specific symptoms in particular populations, often leading to inappropriate differences in diagnoses of specific illnesses in those populations.

Racial Bias and Racialization in Mental Health Policy and Research

The fact that mental health leaders have held to the belief that they can be objective and not bound by culture has repeatedly led to harm against groups that are racially and ethnically oppressed. Consider the work of policy makers, psychiatrists, and mental health advocates working with President Lyndon Johnson throughout the 1960s to combat the war on poverty. In seeking to understand the mental health and intellectual differences among poor and Black families, mental health experts advanced a *cultural deprivation theory* built on a seemingly race-neutral and colorblind framework (Raz 2013). These specialists worked to reframe more overtly racist beliefs of *racial inferiority* into more progressive views of *racial disadvantage* by focusing on what these communities lacked. In regard to cognitive and personal development, cultural deprivation theory argued that racially disadvantaged children lacked maternal nurturing and adequate verbal communication during development, often due to their mothers' deficiencies. These maternal deficiencies included "sensory defects, deficiencies of strength, energy or physical resources, as well as apathy, depression, excessive lability, and marked irritability or hostility" (Raz 2013, pp. 26–27).

Developments in the natural and behavioral sciences during the mid-twentieth century influenced cultural deprivation theory. During the 1950s, scientists at McGill University developed sensory deprivation experiments, which measured the effects of reduced sensory input and social isolation on perceptual disturbances and cognitive deficits (Raz 2011). Scientists used sensory deprivation theory to explain common psychiatric conditions such as confusion and disorientation in hospitalized patients with extended stays and transient psychosis in patients with reduced visual stimuli after ophthalmic surgery. At the same time, noted psychoanalyst John Bowlby developed the term *maternal deprivation* to describe decreased maternal interaction and social isolation during child development (Raz 2011). Similarly, cultural deprivation argued that children who were racially and socioeconomically disadvantaged were more prone to malnourishment, prematurity, adverse health conditions, and inadequate cultural experiences necessary for normal psychological development. Thus, mental health practitioners fastened ideas of maternal and sensory deprivation into theories of social and cultural deprivation to explain developmental psychopathology (Raz 2011).

Explicitly, cultural deprivation theory held that individuals from socially and economically disadvantaged backgrounds lacked the resources necessary to foster adequate psychological well-being. These disadvantaged groups lacked proper psychological development due to their historical oppression, resulting in family structures that lacked cohesion and organization (Fernando 2017; Raz 2013). Cultural deprivation theory drew heavily from *The Mark of Oppression: A Psychosocial Study of the American Negro* (Kardiner and Ovesey 1951). In this psychodynamic case analysis of 25 African Americans, Kardiner and Ovesey (1951) argued that cultural deprivation, less family cohesion, disorganization, and racial discrimination resulted in "depressed-self-esteem" and "self-hatred," which negatively affected Black psychological development (Fernando 2017, p. 65). It is important to note that Kardiner and Ovesey (1951) understood their well-intentioned efforts as racially neutral and progressive, aimed at removing overt forms of racism and discrimination from the scientific discourse. They hoped to illustrate that racial differences are not intrinsic to people who are racially and ethnically oppressed. Kardiner and Ovesey's belief that they could nullify the effect of race merely by espousing their views as race neutral led them to assume their experience of the dominant culture as normative. They did not recognize cultural diversity and the structural causes of racial disadvantage. Policy makers responded in turn by increasing eligibility criteria for low-income families to help them develop as "role models" for their children "to teach them the importance of a good work ethic" (Raz 2013, p. 169). As Raz (2013) argued, "by championing middle-class and wealthy mothers who choose to stay at home to raise their children while simultaneously calling for eligibility criteria that require low-income mothers of young toddlers to work to receive public assistance" (p. 169), policy makers and reformers reinforced normative ideas of cultural deprivation and pathologized the systems of poverty and racial disadvantage that they sought to mitigate.

Although these experts were reacting in good faith to an earlier period of more explicit racism, their approach also was problematic. The explicit goal was to foster a system that minimized the impact and influence of race on individuals, but their approach achieved the opposite effect. Psychology, psychoanalysis, and child development research provided the theoretical foundation for these dominant ideas, yet the scholars and scientists who espoused these ideas failed to recognize that the assessments they made about Black families were unable to account for the "subtle racisms...that assumed that white families and white people were the norm" (Fernando 2017, p. 67). Rather than getting rid of race in their proclamation of a race-neutral framework, they blinded themselves to their implicit biases regarding Black families. In effect, cultural deprivation theory inadvertently pathologized poverty and blamed racially oppressed families for their shortcomings rather than addressing the underlying issues and social structures that explained these inequities.

The example of cultural deprivation theory growing out of the federal "War on Poverty" initiatives represents an attempt to deflect from overtly racist beliefs of racial inferiority to more class-based notions of racial disadvantage. Mental health leaders' adoption of race neutrality and color-blindness as a means to remove the influence of race and racism from social structures was an overly simplistic view that proved to be harmful to people who are racially and ethnically oppressed by pathologizing the poverty built into the very systems in which they live. This example underscores the importance of recognizing the causes and consequences of structural racism in medical theory and practice.

Future Directions for Combating Structural Racism

Structural frameworks and interventions are often underemphasized in traditional psychiatric and mental health training rooted in biopsychosocial interventions and cultural competency. A Robert Wood Johnson Foundation survey found that although 85% of sampled primary care physicians believed that social disparities negatively impact the health of all individuals, they lacked confidence in their ability to meet those needs (Goldstein and Holmes 2011; Metzl and Hansen 2014). Knowledge of structural causes of disease is an essential requirement for mental health care practice. Thus, psychiatric and mental health training should incorporate these perspectives to enable mental health professionals to provide more structurally and culturally informed care and systems of care. Scholars have proposed several frameworks for structural competence to combat structural racism in mental health, which involve identifying and questioning existing structures (Metzl and Hansen 2014, 2018; Metzl and Roberts 2014) (Table 4–1).

Structural racism and discrimination shape the lived experiences and mental life of racially, ethnically, and experientially oppressed populations. Although there is general public consensus decrying the existence of racist attitudes and policies, systems of racism and discrimination persist in U.S. society. From explicit race-based thinking to the unintended, harmful consequences of race-neutral thought, structural racism has impacted the medical and mental health professions explicitly. Understanding the role that race and social structures play in mental health care may help disentangle the role of structural racism and, more effectively, holistically address mental health care for all oppressed individuals.

TABLE 4–1. Frameworks for combating structural racism in mental health

1. Consider social and structural etiologies of disease associations while questioning assumptions about race and biological difference

2. Utilize social sciences and humanities disciplines to interrogate how racism is embedded not only in individual experiences but also within institutional structures

3. Understand the history of race, race-based thinking, and liberal activism in addressing structural racism

4. Work in collaborative settings with other mental health professionals to serve the needs of racially oppressed and vulnerable populations

5. Implement fair hiring policies that help mitigate the societal, economic, and health impacts of practices that disproportionately limit socioeconomic opportunities for racially and ethnically oppressed persons

6. Promote diversity and inclusion such that racially, ethnically, and experientially oppressed persons are not only represented in various social systems and structures but also leveraged in terms of their influence to promote equity for all individuals

7. Advocate for practical and effective policy interventions to reduce the undue burden on oppressed people across social structures (e.g., prohibiting compulsory disclosure for ex-offenders seeking employment)

Questions for Self-Reflection

1. How has structural racism impacted me? My patients? My peers? My colleagues?
2. Are there ways in which cultural deprivation theory may have influenced the way I was taught or supervised?
3. What are the ways in which thinking in a race-neutral manner could negatively impact my relationships with my patients, peers, supervisors, or staff members?

References

American Psychiatric Association: Diagnostic and Statistical Manual of Mental Disorders, 5th Edition. Arlington, VA, American Psychiatric Association, 2013

Asad AL, Clair M: Racialized legal status as a social determinant of health. Soc Sci Med 199:19–28, 2018

Bailey ZD, Krieger N, Agénor M, et al: Structural racism and health inequities in the USA: evidence and interventions. Lancet 389:1453–1463, 2017

Baker FM, Bell CC: Issues in the psychiatric treatment of African Americans. Psychiatr Serv 50:362–368, 1999

Bayor RH: Another look at "whiteness": The persistence of ethnicity in American life. J Am Ethn Hist 29:13–30, 2009

Bonilla-Silva E: Rethinking racism: toward a structural interpretation. Am Sociol Rev 62:465–480, 1997

Centers for Disease Control and Prevention: Guidelines for Mental Health Screening During the Domestic Medical Examination for Newly Arrived Refugees. Atlanta, GA, Centers for Disease Control and Prevention, 2012. Available at: www.cdc.gov/immigrantrefugeehealth/guidelines/domestic/mental-health-screening-guidelines.html. Accessed April 25, 2020.

Centers for Disease Control and Prevention: Technical Instructions for Physical or Mental Disorders With Associated Harmful Behaviors and Substance-Related Disorders for Panel Physicians. Atlanta, GA, Centers for Disease Control and Prevention, 2017. Available at: www.cdc.gov/immigrantrefugeehealth/exams/ti/panel/mental-panel-technical-instructions.html. Accessed April 25, 2020.

Council of National Psychological Associations for the Advancement of Ethnic Minority Interests. Testing and Assessment With Persons and Communities of Color. Edited by Leong FTL, Park YS. Washington, DC, American Psychological Association, 2016

Doyle D: Psychiatry and Racial Liberalism in Harlem, 1936–1968. Rochester, NY, University of Rochester Press, 2016

Dudley RG: African Americans and the criminal justice system, in Black Mental Health: Patients, Providers, and Systems. Edited by Griffith EEH, Jones BE, Stewart AJ. Washington, DC, American Psychiatric Publishing, 2019, pp 65–76

Escarce JJ, Morales LS, Rumbaut RG: The health status and health behaviors of Hispanics, in Hispanics and the Future of America. Edited by Tienda M, Mitchell F. Washington, DC, National Academies Press, 2006, pp 376–377

Fernando S: Institutional Racism in Psychiatry and Clinical Psychology: Race Matters in Mental Health. New York, Springer International, 2017

Frueh BC, Hamner MB, Bernat JA, et al: Racial differences in psychotic symptoms among combat veterans with PTSD. Depress Anxiety 16:157–161, 2002

Garcini LM, Peña JM, Galvan T, et al: Mental disorders among undocumented Mexican immigrants in high-risk neighborhoods: prevalence, comorbidity, and vulnerabilities. J Consult Clin Psychol 85:927–936, 2017

Gee GC, Ford CL: Structural racism and health inequities: old issues, new directions. Du Bois Rev 8:115–132, 2011

Giddens A, Duneier M, Appelbaum RP, Carr D: Introduction to Sociology. New York, WW Norton, 2008

Goldstein D, Holmes J: 2011 Physicians' Daily Life Report. Chicago, IL, Harris Interactive, November 15, 2011. Available at: www.issuelab.org/resources/12550/12550.pdf. Accessed April 25, 2020.

Hatzenbuehler ML, Prins SJ, Flake M, et al: Immigration policies and mental health morbidity among Latinos: a state-level analysis. Soc Sci Med 174:169–178, 2017

Hutton HE, Miner MH, Blades JR, Langfeldt VC: Ethnic differences on the MMPI Overcontrolled-Hostility scale. J Pers Assess 58:260–268, 1992

Kandel WA: Permanent Employment-Based Immigration and the Per-Country Ceiling. Washington, DC, Congressional Research Service, December 21, 2018. Available at: https://crsreports.congress.gov/product/pdf/R/R45447. Accessed April 25, 2020.

Kardiner A, Ovesey L: The Mark of Oppression: A Psychosocial Study of the American Negro. New York, WW Norton, 1951

Klonoff EA, Landrine H, Ullman JB: Racial discrimination and psychiatric symptoms among blacks. Cultur Divers Ethnic Minor Psychol 5:329–339, 1999

Kugelmass H: "Sorry, I'm not accepting new patients": an audit study of access to mental health care. J Health Soc Behav 57:168–183, 2016

Link BG, Phelan J: Social conditions as fundamental causes of disease. J Health Soc Behav Special Issue:80–94, 1995

Lopez-Class M, Castro FG, Ramirez AG: Conceptions of acculturation: a review and statement of critical issues. Soc Sci Med 72:1555–1562, 2011

McCreary C, Padilla E: MMPI differences among black, Mexican American, and white male offenders. J Clin Psychol 33:171–177, 1977

Metzl JM, Hansen H: Structural competency: theorizing a new medical engagement with stigma and inequality. Soc Sci Med 103:126–133, 2014

Metzl JM, Hansen H: Structural competency and psychiatry. JAMA Psychiatry 75:115–116, 2018

Metzl JM, Roberts DE: Structural competency meets structural racism: race, politics, and the structure of medical knowledge. AMA J Ethics 16:674–690, 2014

Monk EP: The consequences of "race and color" in Brazil. Soc Probl 63:413–430, 2016

Nichols VC, LeBrón AMW, Pedraza FI: Policing us sick: the health of Latinos in an era of heightened deportations and racialized policing. Pol Sci Polit 51:293–297, 2018

Obermeyer Z, Powers B, Vogeli C, Mullainathan S: Dissecting racial bias in an algorithm used to manage the health of populations. Science 366:447–453, 2019

Painter NI: The History of White People. New York, WW Norton, 2011

Patler C, Pirtle WL: From undocumented to lawfully present: do changes to legal status impact psychological well-being among Latino immigrant young adults? Soc Sci Med 199:39–48, 2018

Raz M: Was cultural deprivation in fact sensory deprivation? Deprivation, retardation, and intervention in the USA. Hist Human Sci 24:51–69, 2011

Raz M: What's Wrong With the Poor? Psychiatry, Race, and the War on Poverty. Chapel Hill, University of North Carolina Press, 2013

U.S. Department of Health and Human Services: Mental Health: Culture, Race, and Ethnicity—A Supplement to Mental Health: A Report of the Surgeon General. Rockville, MD, Substance Abuse and Mental Health Services Administration, 2001

Wailoo K, Pemberton S: The Troubled Dream of Genetic Medicine: Ethnicity and Innovation in Tay-Sachs, Cystic Fibrosis, and Sickle Cell Disease, Baltimore, MD, Johns Hopkins University Press, 2006

Williams DR, McAdams-Mahmoud A: Racism and mental health: pathways, evidence, and needed research, in Black Mental Health: Patients, Providers, and Systems. Edited by Griffith EEH, Jones BE, Stewart AJ. Washington, DC, American Psychiatric Publishing, 2019, pp 269–281

Williams DR, Mohammed SA: Racism and health I: pathways and scientific evidence. Am Behav Sci 57:1152–1173, 2013

Witherspoon DH, Wooding S, Rogers AR, Marchani EE: Genetic similarities within and between human populations. Genetics 176:351–359, 2007

PART II
SYSTEMS AND STRUCTURES

CHAPTER 5

Social Injustice and the Schooling System

Tiffani Marie, Ph.D.
Brennin Y. Brown, M.D.

Healthy child development is a cornerstone on which human potential is fully realized. Opportunities to identify and build on abilities and strengths are critical for a successful transition from childhood through adolescence to a healthy, productive adulthood. A safe, nurturing educational environment that promotes discovery and understanding—of oneself and one's society—is a foundational social determinant of health because educational attainment is a powerful predictor of numerous health outcomes throughout the life span (Cutler and Lleras-Muney 2006). Schools are uniquely positioned to play a critical role in positive child development. Unfortunately, for many children, schools fail. For these children, school is not a place where they progress; rather, it is one in which they are set on a course replete with inequities. As early as preschool, outcomes in the school environment predict life trajectories in social, economic, and health realms (Reynolds and Ou 2011; Topitzes et al. 2009).

If children receive the free and appropriate education to which they are entitled by law, then school is a place where they understand and develop their potential. If children receive supportive, empathetic responses from school personnel when developmentally appropriate ranges of human emotions are displayed, then school is a place where they learn to use a growing repertoire of adaptive coping skills. If children receive affirming messages about their abilities and stimulating instruction that prepares them for college or the workplace, then school is a place where they can dream of and work toward adult success. However, far too often, school is a place where the path to the full realization of some children's potential is blocked. For far too many young people, school is a place where they are exposed to structural inequities and structural violence and then punished for displaying distress—a place where they are derailed educationally and occupationally.

The educational system (or, more accurately, the *schooling system*, as we refer to it in this chapter) plays a pivotal role in the mental development of children, and it also factors prominently in their utilization of mental health services. Many schools are the primary site for children's mental health care delivery, particularly in communities with limited access to specialized mental health services (Atkins et al. 2017). When community mental health care services *are* available, school staff are characterized as *gateway providers* because of their role in making referrals and linking children to care (Stiffman et al. 2004). In sum, children and families regularly present for mental health treatment because they are affected by their experiences within the school system, referred by the school system, or both. Given that 90% of U.S. children attend public schools (National Center for Education Statistics 2019b), knowledge of the schooling system, including the historical and contemporary contexts for its design and the populations it perpetually fails, is a prerequisite for anyone seeking to understand equity, justice, and mental health issues impacting children.

Regrettably, many mental health professionals and schooling system professionals (e.g., counselors, psychologists, psychiatrists, teachers, principals, researchers) are not fully capable of supporting the youth most negatively impacted by the structural failures of the schooling system. These professionals have gained upward mobility by means of their proximity and conformity to the functions of schools. They are frequently the very people who focus on the outliers, often themselves, who have benefited greatly from schooling, while they neglect the glaring failure of others, a situation that allows for this success. Thus, it is even more critical that these professionals are intentional in reflecting on the historical context and present implications of the schooling system. In this chapter, we examine the interplay between this context; these implications; and the unjust, systematic denial of education and opportunity for entire populations of children.

Historical Context of the U.S. Schooling System

The foundation of American society centers on a belief and investment in education. As early as the Constitutional Convention in 1787, delegates argued over the role of education but agreed on its utility as a primary institution in the formation and future of the country. In the evolution of schools, some U.S. presidents have been more explicit in their relationship to education and its significance. Presidents Lyndon B. Johnson and Ronald Reagan were named *education presidents*, with Johnson suggesting the need for educational projects as a way to eliminate poverty. Johnson's vision for education directly aligned with that of Horace Mann, the American educational reformer and architect of schools, who described education as the "great equalizer" (Mann 1848/1979).

Although consensus surrounding the *need* for an institution of schooling has been a part of the fabric of American society since its inception, its *purpose* has been widely contested. Some education researchers have suggested that the purpose of U.S. schooling is to promote assimilation and instill moral values and ideologies of nationalism within citizens. Others have suggested that schools function to provide economic stability for all who participate. Historian Joel Spring (1989) suggested that the economic, political, and social facets of schooling all function as a means of improving social conditions and cultivating well-educated, trained citizens to contribute successfully to a democratic society. In contrast, other education researchers (Dumas 2014; Duncan-Andrade and Morrell 2008) have highlighted the social inequities reproduced by schools. Bowles and Gintis (1976) suggested that the U.S. schooling system is responsible for the reproduction of patterns of social class and racial inequities.

Examining the history of U.S. schooling system policy highlights this reproduction of inequity. The 1642 Massachusetts Bay Colony laws ensured that only wealthy, white, free young men could have access to education (Ensign 1921). The 1785 Continental Congress Survey of the Northwest Territory influenced the creation of townships and land grant universities through the usurping of Indigenous land (Carstensen 1988; Key 1996). In the early 1800s, schools followed the Lancasterian model, which emphasized the discipline and obedience that factory owners sought in their workers (Jeynes 2007; Upton 1996). Educational policy in the 1830s criminalized access to literacy for Black people (Monaghan 1998; Woodson 1933). The 1851 Massachusetts Compulsory Laws emphasized the "civilizing" of immigrant children to prevent social upheaval (Bandiera et al. 2019). Beginning in 1860, schools worked openly with the U.S. government to forcefully dislocate Indigenous children—as young as 4 years old—from homes, languages, and cultures to attend boarding schools. This process is documented as a federally mandated educational policy that sought to "kill the Indian...and save the man" (Adams 1995, p. 52). Thus, the history of U.S. schools is not of realizing society's collective potential but of perpetuating its hierarchies.

The Schooling System's Place in Perpetuating Social Hierarchies

With this historical foundation, the ensuing educational policies and practices normed within schools positioned schools as exceptionally impactful, insidious, and persistent sites for the reproduction of social inequity. Unquestionably, more than two centuries of degrading and dislocating educational policies can have tremendous impacts on children's mental health and educational outcomes. Theoretical frameworks in the educational literature seek to explain why certain groups have not been able to utilize U.S. schooling to learn their way out of poverty en masse. Namely, poor Black and Latinx youth have dominated education theory as two demographic groups that have been the most unsuccessful within U.S. schools (Duncan-Andrade 2009; Ladson-Billings 1998). The term *achievement gap* has been applied to inequities in educational outcomes (Ladson-Billings 2006), with research focusing on the inability of these youth to successfully progress within schools. Education theory has provided frameworks surrounding grit and perseverance, which are characterized as tools for young people to better navigate the toxicities (i.e., negative social determinants of mental health that interfere with successful learning) in their everyday lives that may compromise their engagement and overall successes within schools. Missing from these approaches is an analysis of the toxicity that *is* U.S. schooling.

Some educational research conceptualizes student failure as a result of individual pathological behavior (Duckworth 2016; Love 2019). This work is emblematic of the more prevalent and highly problematic conversation regarding educational outcomes—the false narrative that success is within everyone's reach. As it stands, if all of our youth were successful, by the defining terms of schools (i.e., honor roll students who perform well on entrance exams), we could not possibly have enough capacity in our colleges and universities to serve them. That is, within our school system with our society as currently configured, someone has to fail (Duncan-Andrade and Morrell 2008). This perpetuates the stratification in our society, which relies on a foundation of the working class to support the very few who will have access to higher education and other forms of upward mobility. As a result, the schooling system has become an important sorting mechanism for systemic inequity, subjecting Black and Latinx children in particular to structural violence.

Adversities of Black Students Within the Schooling System

Educational research has documented numerous studies of Black students' adversities within schools. These experiences are often recorded as perpetual and disproportionate rates of underachievement, dropouts, suspensions, expulsions, and referrals to special education (Akom 2003; Duncan-Andrade and Morrell 2008). However, these data frame the issue from only one perspective. Other research on educational outcomes of Black students within schools accounts for the disproportionate physical and mental violence that Black youth endure, including dilapidated and underresourced schools (Kozol 2012), ongoing bodily harassment (Wun 2016), surveillance (Farmer 2010), and attacks on their self-esteem and self-worth (Crenshaw et al. 2015; Dumas 2014). Together, these research outcomes promote a more balanced and robust understanding of the disenfranchisement and mental trauma of Black children within schools. They extend beyond theories that are concerned solely with academic achievement toward a model that seeks to identify and eradicate attacks on the minds, bodies, and spirits of Black children.

Social Reproduction of Black Suffering

Although some researchers disregard the relationship between race, socioeconomic status, and social stratification, conceptualizing Black suffering as individual pathology (Clark 1989), others argue that failure within Black schools is by design (Duncan-Andrade and Morrell 2008). For example, many school district budgets rely on property taxes for school resources. As a result, wealthier, predominantly white communities have access to greater monetary resources, cultivating more robust per-pupil spending. Although some states, such as California, have capped per-pupil public spending, resulting in some improvement in funding inequity from public dollars, such policies do not prevent private organizations in wealthier communities, such as parent-teacher associations, from raising thousands to millions of dollars each year (Goldstein 2017). Additionally, many of the poorest districts in the country serve the highest concentrations of Black students; these schools in turn receive far fewer resources than all other schools (National Equity Atlas 2020). Schools then reproduce social realities in which individiuals with the most continue to have the most, and those with the least continue to be pathologized as the cause of their own disenfranchisement (Dumas and Ross 2016).

Neoliberal Explanations of Black Suffering in Education

Neoliberal explanations of Black suffering have recently gained traction within the field of education. Since the 1980s, such explanations have served to shift the national conversation away from one that engages race. This approach presumes that racism is no longer a hindrance to equality; thus, those who do not experience upward mobility are believed to have failed on their own, particularly as a result of their inability to work hard enough (Dumas and Ross 2016). Neoliberalism is evident in the narratives surrounding charter schools (i.e., public schools governed by a private board rather than the state board of education). This narrative publicizes rags-to-riches approaches to education (Wells et al. 1999), celebrating outliers within Black communities who defy the odds and can gain access to upward mobility. Often, these communities are characterized by structural violence in the form of poverty, mass incarceration, and lack of healthy food options and green space. These acts of structural violence are neatly framed as obstacles and rarely acknowledged as what they are in reality—effective instruments of oppression.

The charter school educational model, greatly influenced by neoliberal theories, emphasizes grit and delayed gratification as viable means of upward mobility for anyone who works hard enough (Baldridge 2014; Dumas and Ross 2016). Research suggests that neoliberal approaches to education center myths of meritocracy while leaving unchallenged the need for failure within a demanding and awaiting capitalist market (Akom 2003). This is an effective method of overestimating the power of the individual and underestimating the power of structural inequities (Jones and Nisbett 1971). Furthermore, these schools are often staffed by inexperienced teachers and characterized by a high degree of teacher turnover. Teachers use their time serving disadvantaged children as a stepping-stone to secure advanced jobs in social work, medicine, and the juvenile justice system, leaving vulnerable students behind (Labaree 2010).

Societal Coherence Through Black Suffering

Schools are the most impactful and longitudinal iteration of the structural racism that started with enslavement and colonization. Because laws now prohibit overt physical degradation, white supremacists can no longer victimize Black bodies with direct physical violence (e.g., lynchings). The legal system—whose very language of justice, fairness, and equality is laden with hypocrisy and exclusivity—does not have such consistent, far-reaching access to Black bodies. In a country with compulsory education in which 90% of students attend public schools, the schooling system has become the primary institution, across the longest span of time, that inflicts the greatest form of structural violence—the norming of a population's dehumanization (National Center for Education Statistics 2019b).

In 1933, Carter G. Woodson acknowledged the role of schools as a primary institution responsible for the reproduction of Black suffering:

> As another has well said, to handicap a student by teaching him that his black face is a curse and that his struggle to change his condition is hopeless is the worst sort of lynching. It kills one's aspirations and dooms him to vagabondage and crime. Is it strange, then, that the friends of truth and the promoters of freedom have not risen up against the present propaganda in the schools and crushed it. This crusade is much more important than the anti-lynching movement, because there would be no lynching if it did not start in the schoolroom. (Woodson 1933, p. 24)

It would be audacious to point to images of Black people who were victims of lynching in the mid-nineteenth century and blame them for their *own* oppression. However, when we refuse to acknowledge that the U.S. schooling project perpetuates inequality, we are, in effect, blaming students for their oppression. The problem is not the struggling Black student. The problem is any system that positions the student to fail, any system that depends on and profiteers from this degradation. Society's refusal to confront the historical and present structural violence of the U.S. schooling system only serves to increase Black suffering.

Adversities of Latinx Students Within the Schooling System

Black and Latinx students' experiences of adversities within the schooling system often intersect. In fact, study outcomes for Latinx students almost mirror those of Black students around issues of underachievement, dropouts, suspensions and expulsions, and even recommendations for special education (de Brey et al. 2019; Noguera 2003). However, research differs in representations of Latinx students' school experiences related to citizenship and language.

[Righteous] Mistrust of U.S. Schooling

A sociopolitical historical read of Latinx people's experience in the United States would justify Mexican American distrust toward U.S. institutions.

Extensive data document U.S. imperialism in Mexico. Although these histories of imperialism are long-standing, a potential starting point of this turmoil is the 1848 Treaty of Guadalupe Hidalgo, which ended the Mexican-American War. Some historical accounts of the war highlight the imperialist intentions of an emerging U.S. society. They depicted Mexican people as noble, patriotic, and courageous in the defense of their humanity and lands (Acuña 1988; Zinn 1995). Some historians even suggest that the U.S. urgency around the war went beyond an interest in conquering land and encompassed rage toward Mexicans who refused to support the enslavement of African people (Acuña 1988).

However, the emerging narratives of the war were shaped by the conquerors—and then disseminated through U.S. history classes. Many accounts of noble Mexican soldiers were omitted from these lessons. Instead, Mexicans were characterized as defeated, conquered people, dregs even, who lacked the strength and unity to defend themselves from a powerful U.S. army (Acuña 1988). Adjacent to these representations were images of Mexican people as lazy and passive. These one-sided historical accounts are emblematic of the history taught within U.S. schools. For Latinx youth attending U.S. schools, particularly those youth with an awareness of U.S. imperialism, it can be difficult to learn in such a Eurocentric space.

Educational researcher Angela Valenzuela (1999) suggests that "real learning is difficult to sustain in an atmosphere rife with mistrust" (p. 5). Her work highlights the subtractive nature of U.S. schooling for Latinx youth, referring to how it intentionally detaches Latinx youth from their culture, language, and ties to history. She argues that a prerequisite for the academic success of Latinx youth is the denial of themselves, their histories, and their cultural practices. In this context, underachievement for many Latinx youth is reflective of resistance to a subtractive culture. She adds,

> Before dismissing urban, U.S.-born youth as lazy underachievers, it behooves researchers and practitioners to first examine school's role in fostering poor academic performance. Bringing schools into sharper focus...reveals that U.S.-born youth are neither inherently antischool nor oppositional. They oppose a schooling process that disrespects them; they oppose not education, but *schooling*. (Valenzuela 1999, p. 5)

U.S. schooling's subtractive practices have led to the underachievement of Latinx youth, the second-largest demographic adversely impacted by dropouts for over a decade (National Center for Education Statistics 2019a; Valenzuela 2005). Conversely, Valenzuela looks to education (or *educación*, as she refers to it) for the types of enriching practice that engages familial customs, morality, and communal sensibilities. There have been countless educators who have engaged such life-affirming pedagogical practices within schools, yet they have faced extreme opposition (Duncan-Andrade and Morrell 2008). The opposition to their success, particularly with Latinx youth, reflects a tremendous gap between the rhetoric and the reality of the U.S. schooling system.

Neoliberalism and Latinx U.S. School Achievement

Neoliberal policies have had a disproportionate adverse impact on Latinx youth and their schooling experiences. Martinez (2016) argues that neoliberal policies and practices have contributed to drastic funding deficits directly leading to programmatic cuts in K–12 bilingual education and other educational supports. Additionally, the structural responses to Latinx achievement in schools are illustrative of the divide between the rhetoric and the reality of neoliberal policies. As previously noted, neoliberal educational policies often advocate for character traits encompassing grit, delayed gratification, critical thinking, and hard work, yet U.S. leadership has not responded favorably when Latinx groups have exhibited these traits.

Consider the case of Jaime Escalante, a mathematics teacher in the Los Angeles Unified School District, serving primarily Latinx youth. Realizing that his pedagogical interventions were becoming increasingly informed by his Latinx students' low mathematical skills and high scholastic needs, Escalante developed a new approach, which focused on teaching a culturally relevant curriculum (Ladson-Billings 1998). His method both acknowledged students' resistance toward subtractive schooling and drew from students' internal reservoir of cultural assets. Years into Escalante's math intervention, academic achievement improved, and he developed a mathematics program that introduced Advanced Placement (AP) Calculus to students who had previously been labeled "unteachable." At the height of Escalante's career, his Latinx students were passing the AP Calculus test at rates much higher than those of students in neighboring wealthy communities such as Beverly Hills. One year, more than 80% of Escalante's students passed the exam. As a result, his students were accused of cheating, were investigated by government officials, and were required to retake the exam—which they passed. Before his intervention, Escalante's Latinx students were judged for their resistance to schools; however, when they became engaged and excelled in response to his intervention, their character was questioned. This response laid bare that these students had defied the system's actual design, with its underlying expectation that *these* students were not supposed to succeed. When these students *do* succeed, they are routinely accused of cheating and often asked to retake examinations.

Through the vehicle of schooling, race is used to stratify children in a system in which someone has to lose. The realities that Jaime Escalante's students and other Latinx youth experience in U.S. schools are indicative of the reproductive power of social class and racial hierarchies. Latinx and Black youth are often aware of these realities and resist the predictability of schooling in various ways (Kohl 1995). Such "willed not-learning" reflects young people's courageous agency against a structure that compromises their humanity (Kohl 1995). Instead of valuing the critical nature of young people's resistance to schooling, the adults bringing these children for mental health evaluations tend to focus solely on the *maladaptive* behavior. In this context, this behavior may be conceptualized as individual pathology rather than recognized as the socioemotional product of an oppressive system. Youth anger, disengagement, or hopelessness in response to the reproductive nature of schooling is rarely understood as an outcome of the dehumanization and educational neglect that these youth experience.

Ultimately, U.S. schools were neither created nor reformed to promote the universal success of Black or Latinx youth. An examination of the schooling system's origin makes clear its true mandate—to sustain the wealthy and reproduce class inequities for individuals who are poor and nonwhite (Anyon 1980; Duncan-Andrade and Morrell 2008). When Black and Latinx youth were eventually granted access to U.S. schools, the well-oiled machine consistently functioned to reproduce class and racial hierarchies in the form of schools that were highly racially and economically segregated and in the context of a persistent and increasingly widening racial income gap (Richmond 2012). Thus, the theories, data, and examples reviewed in this volume and elsewhere suggest that educational failures are not *by accident*—they are *by design* (Duncan-Andrade and Morrell 2008).

Conclusion

For U.S. schools to shift from sites of social reproduction toward sites of social transformation, the individuals who maintain these spaces—policy makers, theorists, and researchers who often have a stated desire for youth to have better access to achieving purpose-driven lives—must courageously and intentionally acknowledge and grapple with the unfiltered history of this country. Mental health professionals have a role to play, too. With expertise in development, identity formation, and trauma, and with the social standing that comes with being highly educated professionals, clinicians who learn about these issues are uniquely equipped to advocate for children by helping parents, teachers, and the broader society contextualize the children's symptoms of distress. Educational theorist W.E.B. DuBois (1994) argues that to remedy the problems of today, we must turn a keen eye toward their origins, acknowledging hard historical truths so that today's students can benefit from the lessons contained therein.

Many of the architects of U.S. schools articulated a vision for equality and upward mobility for all, while at the same time investing in the enslavement and subjugation of Black, Indigenous, and Latinx people. It makes sense, then, that these contradictions were woven into the fabric of U.S. schooling. Society may profess a desire for equity while engaging in practices that perpetuate stability for very few at the expense of others. These truths have often been absent or minimized in conversations on educational policy and school reform. Both educational policy decision makers and child and adolescent mental health professionals must bear the discomfort of learning from young people most impacted by the toxins inherent in U.S. schooling. This is the first step in moving toward the types of thinking and discussions and ultimately the types of policies and practices that can truly transform society. Moving forward, if the rhetoric of the U.S. school system is to match the reality of its students' experiences, leaders at all levels must engage in profound acts of truth seeking and initiate radical reform.

Questions for Self-Reflection

1. What was my personal schooling experience like when I was growing up? How might this be different from the experiences of the patients I serve?
2. What assumptions do I make about children who are not academically engaged? How might a lack of academic engagement be conceptualized as a structural issue rather than an individual issue?
3. What do I know about the educational outcomes by zip codes in the communities I serve?

References

Acuña R: Occupied America, 3rd Edition. New York, HarperCollins, 1988

Adams DW: Education for Extinction: American Indians and the Boarding School Experience. Lawrence, University Press of Kansas, 1995

Akom AA: Reexamining resistance as oppositional behavior: the Nation of Islam and the creation of a black achievement ideology. Sociol Educ 76:305–325, 2003

Anyon J: Social class and the hidden curriculum of work. J Educ 162:67–92, 1980

Atkins MS, Cappella E, Shernoff ES, et al: Schooling and children's mental health: realigning resources to reduce disparities and advance public health. Annu Rev Clin Psychol 13:123–147, 2017

Baldridge BJ: Relocating the deficit: reimagining black youth in neoliberal times. Am Educ Res J 3:440–472, 2014

Bandiera O, Mohnen M, Rasul I, Viarengo M: Nation-building through compulsory schooling during the age of mass migration. Econ J 129:62–109, 2019

Bowles S, Gintis H: Schooling in Capitalist America: Educational Reform and the Contradictions of Economic Life. New York, Basic Books, 1976

Carstensen V: Patterns on the American land. Publius 18:31–39, 1988

Clark KB: Dark Ghetto: Dilemmas of Social Power, 2nd Edition. Middletown, CT, Wesleyan University Press, 1989

Crenshaw K, Ocen P, Nanda J: Black Girls Matter: Pushed Out, Overpoliced, and Underprotected. New York, Center for Intersectionality and Social Policy Studies, Columbia University, 2015

Cutler DM, Lleras-Muney A: Education and Health: Evaluating Theories and Evidence. Ann Arbor, MI, National Bureau of Economic Research, 2006

de Brey C, Musu L, McFarland J, et al: Status and Trends in the Education of Racial and Ethnic Groups 2018. Washington, DC, U.S. Department of Education, 2019

DuBois WEB: The Souls of Black Folk. North Chelmsford, MA, Courier, 1994

Duckworth A: Grit: The Power of Passion and Perseverance. New York, Scribner, 2016

Dumas MJ: "Losing an arm": schooling as a site of black suffering. Race Ethn Educ 17:1–29, 2014

Dumas MJ, Ross KM: "Be real black for me": imagining BlackCrit in education. Urban Educ 51:415–442, 2016

Duncan-Andrade JM: Note to educators: hope required when growing roses in concrete. Harv Educ Rev 79:181–194, 2009

Duncan-Andrade JM, Morrell E: The Art of Critical Pedagogy: Possibilities for Moving From Theory to Practice in Urban Schools. New York, Peter Lang, 2008

Ensign FC: Compulsory School Attendance and Child Labor. Iowa City, IA, Athens Press, 1921

Farmer S: Criminality of black youth in inner-city schools: "moral panic," moral imagination, and moral formation. Race Ethn Educ 3:367–381, 2010

Goldstein D: PTA gift for someone else's child? A touchy subject in California. New York Times, April 9, 2017

Jeynes WH: American Educational History: School, Society, and the Common Good. Thousand Oaks, CA, Sage, 2007

Jones EE, Nisbett RE: The Actor and the Observer; Divergent Perceptions of the Causes of Behavior. Morristown, NJ, General Learning Press, 1971

Key S: Economics or education: the establishment of American land-grant universities. J Higher Educ 67:196–220, 1996

Kohl HR: I Won't Learn From You, and Other Thoughts on Creative Maladjustment. New York, New Press, 1995

Kozol J: Savage Inequalities: Children in America's Schools. New York, Broadway Books, 2012

Labaree D: Teach for America and teacher ed: heads they win, tails we lose. J Teach Educ 61:48–55, 2010

Ladson-Billings G: Just what is critical race theory and what's it doing in a nice field like education? Int J Qual Stud Educ 11:7–24, 1998

Ladson-Billings G: From the achievement gap to the education debt: understanding achievement in U.S. schools. Educ Res 35:3–12, 2006

Love BL: We Want to Do More Than Survive: Abolitionist Teaching and the Pursuit of Educational Freedom. Boston, MA, Beacon Press, 2019

Mann H: Twelfth annual report to the Massachusetts Board of Education (1848), in The Republic and the School: Horace Mann and the Education of Free Men. Edited by Cremin LA. New York, Teachers College Press, 1979, pp 79–112

Martinez RO: The impact of neoliberalism on Latinos. Lat Stud 14:11–32, 2016

Monaghan EJ: Reading for the enslaved, writing for the free: reflections on liberty and literacy. Proc Am Antiq Soc 108:309, 1998

National Center for Education Statistics: Fast Facts: Dropout Rates. Washington, DC, National Center for Education Statistics, 2019a. Available at: https://nces.ed.gov/fastfacts/display.asp?id=16. Accessed May 10, 2020.

National Center for Education Statistics: Fast Facts: Public School Choice Programs. Washington DC, National Center for Education Statistics, 2019b. Available at: https://nces.ed.gov/fastfacts/display.asp?id=6#:~:text=Also%20in%202016%2C%20some%2020,percent%20attended%20a%20private%20school. Accessed September 6, 2020.

National Equity Atlas: Indicators: School Poverty. Oakland, CA, PolicyLink, 2020. Available at: https://nationalequityatlas.org/indicators/School_poverty. Accessed May 10, 2020.

Noguera PA: The trouble with black boys: the role and influence of environmental and cultural factors on the academic performance of African American males. Urban Educ 38:431–459, 2003

Reynolds AJ, Ou SR: Paths of effects from preschool to adult well-being: a confirmatory analysis of the child-parent center program. Child Dev 82:555–582, 2011

Richmond E: Schools are more segregated today than during the late 1960s. Atlantic Magazine, June 11, 2012. Available at: www.theatlantic.com/national/archive/2012/06/schools-are-more-segregated-today-than-during-the-late-1960s/258348. Accessed May 7, 2020.

Spring JH: The Sorting Machine Revisited: National Educational Policy Since 1945. New York, Longman, 1989

Stiffman AR, Pescosolido B, Cabassa LJ: Building a model to understand youth service access: the gateway provider model. Ment Health Serv Res 6:189–198, 2004

Topitzes J, Godes O, Mersky JP, et al: Educational success and adult health: findings from the Chicago Longitudinal Study. Prev Sci 10:175–195, 2009

Upton D: Lancasterian schools, republican citizenship, and the spatial imagination in early nineteenth-century America. Journal of the Society of Architectural Historians 55:238–253, 1996

Valenzuela A: Subtractive Schooling: U.S.-Mexican Youth and the Politics of Caring. New York, State University New York Press, 1999

Valenzuela A (ed): Leaving Children Behind: How "Texas-Style" Accountability Fails Latino Youth. Albany, State University of New York Press, 2005

Wells AS, Lopez A, Scott J, Holme JJ: Charter schools as postmodern paradox: rethinking social stratification in an age of deregulated school choice. Harv Educ Rev 2:172–205, 1999

Woodson CG: The Mis-Education of the Negro. Washington, DC, Associated Publishers, 1933

Wun C: Against captivity: black girls and school discipline policies in the afterlife of slavery. Educ Policy 30:171–196, 2016

Zinn H: A People's History of the United States: 1492–Present, 2nd edition. New York, Harper Collins, 1995

CHAPTER 6

Social Injustice and the Child Welfare System

Melissa D. Carter, J.D.
Courtney L. McMickens, M.D., M.P.H., M.H.S.

The family is the basic organizing unit of society. It is an institution arising from intimate relationships—those between spouses or partners, children and their parents, and extended family networks—connected by biology, created by law through marriage or adoption or formed by choice. Values, traditions, culture, and behavioral norms are transmitted to future generations through these relationships, and legal rights and obligations are assigned and fulfilled. The family is also the foundation for the psychological, physical, and emotional development of children—first, in terms of providing basic needs and protection and also in terms of modeling relationship engagement and teaching prosocial behavior. The individual and societal importance of family, however structured, cannot be completely separated.

The significance of the family as a sociolegal institution is reflected in the scope of constitutional protection afforded to it. The U.S. Supreme Court has repeatedly recognized a "private realm of family life which the state cannot enter" (*Pierce v. Society of Sisters* 1925) and a corresponding liberty interest in the parent-child relationship protected by the Fourteenth

Amendment (*Meyer v. Nebraska* 1923). The right of the family to be free from government intervention is not absolute, however. The state has the power—and some might say the duty—to intervene in the family to protect a child from abuse or neglect (*Prince v. Massachusetts* 1944). This authority to intrude on family privacy and limit family autonomy is exercised routinely by state child welfare systems that receive, investigate, and respond to reports of suspected child maltreatment. The child welfare system is perhaps best understood with reference to its familiar programmatic features: child protection, foster care, and adoption. It is an extensively regulated system that functions at the local, state, and federal levels through a financing and service delivery model designed to promote the safety, permanency, and well-being of children and the general welfare of families with whom the state intervenes. It pursues these goals in seemingly contradictory ways, reflecting the influence of social and political views on the institution of the family.

The child welfare system is, at once, a system of preserving and strengthening families and one of separating families in the name of child protection. It is a system of social welfare through which the government provides aid and assistance to families in need and one of coercive intervention that carries the threat of the permanent destruction of a family. It also is a system that exists for the sake of all children but one that operates in profoundly inequitable ways, particularly as it affects children of color and poor children. Decisions to intervene in families ultimately turn on the judgment of professionals carrying out mandates that are heavily influenced by historical, social, economic, and political views on the appropriate function of family and the proper role of government. In this way, structural racism and classism affect which families are afforded privacy and which are subject to government surveillance and intrusion. The measure of privacy afforded to families reflects the traditional concept of the American *family ideal* and the deeply rooted personal beliefs and experiences, cultural expectations, and social norms about child rearing, family functioning, and parenting standards that accompany it. Those views become enshrined as public policy in laws that reinforce and perpetuate inequalities in system and individual outcomes.

The foundational principle of the child welfare system is that the government bears responsibility for protecting its most vulnerable citizens, chief among them children who are suffering abuse or who require basic care. When examined through a racial lens, that protection does not look the same for Black and Indigenous children as it does for white children (Table 6–1). At present, nearly 438,000 children are in foster care throughout the United States (U.S. Children's Bureau 2019). Of those children, 23% are Black and 2% are American Indian/Alaska Native; however, Black and American Indian/Alaska Native children constitute only 14% and 1% of all children in the U.S. child population, respectively (Annie E. Casey Foundation 2019;

TABLE 6–1. Child welfare statistics by race, fiscal year 2018

Race/ethnicity	Confirmed reports of maltreatment (%)	Involvement in foster care (%)	U.S. child population
American Indian/Alaska Native	1.4	2	1.6
Black or African American	20.5	21	13.7
Asian	0.9	1	9.8
White	44.3	47	50.3
Native Hawaiian/ Pacific Islander	0.2	0	0.3
Unknown	5.1	2	NA
Two or more races	5.2	7	8.4
Hispanic (of any race)	22.4	20	25.5

Note. NA=not available.
Source. U.S. Children's Bureau 2019, 2020.

U.S. Children's Bureau 2019). This overrepresentation of Black and Indigenous children has persisted for decades because of the complex interplay of historical and contemporary effects of racism and poverty.

A discriminatory racial pattern is also documented in studies of service and placement inequities (Hill 2006). These service challenges are illustrated most clearly in the arena of mental health. Families become involved with the child welfare system because of neglect, physical abuse, parental substance abuse, inadequate housing, and parental incarceration or death (U.S. Children's Bureau 2019). Emotional and behavioral symptoms, such as avoidance, defiance, anger, social withdrawal, inattention, or emotional detachment, can be observed in children who have experienced traumatic events. Thus, the fact that children in foster care are 10 times more likely than children in the community to have seen a mental health provider is not surprising (Garland et al. 1996). Common diagnoses among children within the mental health system include conduct disorder, ADHD, PTSD, and mood disorders. Beyond formal diagnoses, however, the psychological toll of trauma, family disruption, and placement in foster care for some children is ever-present. The mental health needs of these children go unmet for various reasons, including lack of dissemination of effective practices, limited funding, difficulty engaging families, and ineffective collaboration between child-serving systems (Garcia et al. 2015). The unavoidable reality is that families of color are subject to more government intervention but are less likely to have their needs adequately addressed. These inequities are deeply rooted in the historical origins of the child welfare system and the societal context of structural vulnerability based on race and class.

The Origin Story of Child Welfare

No account of child protection history in the United States is complete without the story of Mary Ellen Wilson. Grainy black-and-white photos of 9-year-old Mary Ellen with a large gash across her face and bruises and cuts on her arms and legs document the abusive conditions she endured, and the modern child welfare system bears the imprint of her rescue story. As the story goes, Mary Ellen was taken under guardianship in 1866 after her father died in her infancy and her mother surrendered her for adoption (Jalongo 2006). For years, Mary Ellen's guardians routinely beat her and neglected her basic needs until neighbors got the attention of Etta Wheeler, an area mission worker. On investigation of their claims, Wheeler discovered a malnourished, frail, emotionally withdrawn, and physically battered child. Eventually, Wheeler persuaded Henry Bergh, the founder of the American Society for the Prevention of Cruelty to Animals, to intervene on Mary Ellen's behalf. The two quickly obtained court authorization for her removal from the home. The girl was in such poor condition that an observer in court that day wrote, "I saw a child brought in…at the sight of which men wept aloud. And as I looked, I knew I was where the first chapter of children's rights was written" (Jalongo 2006, p. 3). Indeed, Mary Ellen's ordeal is often cited as the origin story for what has become the organized, government-sponsored child welfare system of today.

This legendary narrative of child rescue does not provide a full account of child protection history, however. As more formal child welfare systems developed, Black children were largely excluded from orphanages and foster homes. Billingsley and Giovannoni (1972) published a seminal work that defined the role of institutional racism in the child welfare system's interactions with Black families. In *Children of the Storm: Black Children and American Child Welfare*, they identified three ways in which structural racism has historically been operationalized: negative evaluation of Black families, exclusion of Black families from development of policies and systems, and exclusion of Black families from services and supports (Harris 2014). In southern states, where a large proportion of Black populations resided, the end of slavery in 1863 left Black families impoverished. State-sanctioned segregation, discrimination, and racism continued to permeate every aspect of society, leaving Black families with limited access to jobs, education, and social welfare services (Brice 2017). Black families developed systems of extended family, churches, and social organizations to provide aid for orphaned children or families in need of financial assistance well into the twentieth century, when child welfare services were integrated in the South (Brice 2017; Hill 2004).

Another key historical illustration of the conflictual involvement of family and state intervention along the lines of race and power is the experience of Indigenous families. In the late 1800s, authorities facilitated a movement based on the racist belief that American Indians were "uncivilized" and that American Indian mothers were not adequately assimilated to raise their children properly (Jacobs 2013). This resulted in the separation of thousands of children from their families for decades, from the late nineteenth century into the early twentieth century. Indigenous children were placed in remote boarding schools, leaving generations with no awareness of their native culture, and many Indigenous family structures fractured. This so-called intervention disempowered tribal authority and promoted the family structure of middle-class European American culture as superior. The overrepresentation of Indigenous children in the foster care system has continued, even with the dismantling of boarding school enrollment (Jacobs 2013).

The Entanglement of Child Protection, Poverty, and Race

Historically, poverty has been seen as a threat to the vitality of the family institution. Beginning in the nineteenth century, urbanization exposed the needs of destitute, runaway, and abandoned children in more concentrated and visible ways (Trammell 2009). Prior to a more formalized system, there was a system, largely in the urban northeastern areas, of indentureship and workhouses that were deemed relief for the poor in which impoverished families, including children, would provide services as payment (Brice 2017). Public policy responses focused on the economic conditions of the family and the destabilizing effects of poverty on the life course and well-being of children. Children who were poor were understood to be dependent; their circumstances were not distinct from their state of being. The singular child protection response was to remove the children from their environment. A system of *placing out* emerged as the preferred alternative to the institutionalization of dependent children (Trammell 2009). In this system, dependent children were placed with private families rather than in institutions. Charles Loring Brace and the New York Children's Aid Society are credited with developing the first child relocation model, which served as the genesis for the orphan train movement, a supervised relocation and resettlement strategy (Holt 1994). Between 1854 and 1929, as many as 200,000 children are believed to have been separated from their families via the orphan train movement, and most were never reunited (Trammell 2009).

Over time, provision for dependent children, which had been local and private, increasingly became more organized and eventually shifted to being the responsibility of state government agencies and newly emerging juvenile courts (Myers 2008). The call for a greater governmental role in child protection in order to maintain families arose in part from criticisms of the orphan train movement as lacking oversight and standards for placement. The federal government responded to this call, in part, with the first White House Conference on Dependent Children in 1909. The request for the conference came to President Theodore Roosevelt from former-orphan-turned-lawyer James West and a small group of child rescuers (U.S. Children's Bureau 1967). The recommendations issued after the conference stressed the importance of families, concluding, "Home life is the highest and finest product of civilization.... Children should not be deprived of it except for urgent and compelling reasons. Except in unusual circumstances, the home should not be broken up for reasons of poverty" (U.S. Children's Bureau 1967, p. 4). This belief—that government should protect families by ensuring they receive adequate support during times of major economic shifts—was the impetus for the pursuit of a modern welfare state.

The 1930s ushered in the era of government-sponsored child welfare under an approach that forged an enduring link between economic welfare policy and child welfare policy. The mothers' pension laws in the early 1900s were an initial government response to the needs of poor children. Although designed to support the preservation of families through the provision of financial assistance, such laws typically conditioned eligibility for benefits on a home being found *suitable* or parent-recipients being deemed worthy (Roberts 1999). Without clear standards, implementation turned on subjective notions about the deservingness of a family. As a result, Black and immigrant mothers were excluded from participating or received reduced benefits (Roberts 2002). As part of President Franklin Roosevelt's New Deal, the Social Security Act of 1935 created Aid to Dependent Children (ADC), later renamed Aid to Families with Dependent Children (AFDC). Influenced by the tradition of the mothers' pension law that preceded it, the ADC program provided cash assistance to mothers rearing children with absent or incapacitated fathers (Pelton 1987).

The Social Security Act of 1935 concurrently established the Child Welfare Services Program to provide grants to states to help dependent and neglected children and began the federalization of child protection. The Children's Bureau was authorized "to cooperate with State public-welfare agencies in establishing, extending, and strengthening, in rural areas, public welfare services for the protection and care of homeless, dependent, and neglected children, and children in danger of becoming delinquent" (Social Security Act of 1935). As a matter of policy, state intervention was seen as a necessary tool of economic justice. Still today, state responses to child abuse and neglect are influenced heavily by the availability of federal funding tied to substantive and procedural legal mandates dictating how state child welfare systems should operate. Decades of these federal mandates charted a course for the modern child welfare system based on the archetypal family and the child-rescue philosophy imprinted on the system long ago. In this way, the racially and socially constructed ideology of the family that appears in the early history of child protection and child welfare policy has been carried forward into laws that institutionalize discriminatory patterns of response and family intervention. As a matter of practice, however, the child welfare system expanded governmental reach into the lives of greater numbers of families of color, and public child welfare caseloads began increasing (Roberts 2002). The results are racially disproportionate effects throughout the myriad system touch points within a family.

The effects of poverty confound research examining racial inequities in child maltreatment (Hill 2006). Still, some racial effects appear with relative consistency. Studies find that families of color are more likely to be reported to child protective services, and reports involving families of color are investigated and substantiated at disproportionate rates (Hill 2006). Once removed from their families, minority children remain in foster care longer, and Black children are less likely than white children to be adopted or reunified with their families (Hill 2006). Several theories have been put forward to explain these inequities, each of which speaks to the structural racism and classism that pervade public policies, institutional practices, and system norms:

- Disproportionate and disparate needs of children and families of color, particularly due to higher rates of poverty
- Racial bias and discrimination exhibited by individuals (e.g., caseworkers, mandated and other reporters)
- Child welfare system factors (e.g., lack of resources for families of color, caseworker characteristics) (U.S. Children's Bureau 2016, p. 5)

For the most part, federal child welfare laws have not confronted these individual or systemic factors or attempted to target and correct the root causes of racial and economic inequities in how the system operates. Instead, anchored by historical influences, child welfare laws largely have served to perpetuate the socially constructed family ideal and child-rescue mentality (Table 6–2).

The Child Abuse Prevention and Treatment Act of 1974 (CAPTA), the first federal child welfare legislation, created a framework for a public detection system by providing federal funding to states that had enacted laws providing for the reporting of known or suspected instances of child abuse and neglect. All states had mandatory reporting laws by 1967, prior to CAPTA's enactment, but the availability of federal funding intensified and expanded surveillance of families at the community level, particularly through avenues of social services, education, and health care (Myers 2008). Racial bias and discrimination now had an institutional expression, which manifested as persistent racial disproportionality in child maltreatment victimization rates, meaning the maltreatment report was substantiated or indicated (i.e., highly suspected). In the most recent report on child protective service response, the U.S. Children's Bureau (2020) reported victimization rates for the three races representing the most victims. The pronounced disproportionality of Black children appears when comparing these rates with the racial distributions for all children in the population, which the Children's Bureau reported as 50.3% white, 25.5% Latinx, and 13.7% Black (U.S. Children's Bureau 2020). Evaluation of maltreatment rates shows overall higher rates of reported and substantiated abuse among Black children than white children; among Latinx children, reported rates of abuse were comparatively higher, but substantiated rates were lower (Sedlak et al. 2010).

An expanded detection system and an emphasis on identification of abuse and neglect predictably led to an increase in the nation's foster care system. By 1977, more than 500,000 children were in foster care throughout the United States (Ensign 1989). Policy makers naturally became concerned about the unnecessary removal of children and the lack of oversight of the foster care system generally. A particular injustice was unfolding in the Native American community, as reportedly 25%–35% of Native American children were being removed from their parents for alleged abuse or neglect (Myers 2008). Moreover, children who had been removed from parental custody by the state were lingering in foster care, raising concern about the lack of meaningful efforts to reunify families. In response, Congress enacted the Indian Child Welfare Act of 1978 (ICWA) to protect the integrity of Native American tribes and families. Today, the historical patterns of forced family separation endure. More than four decades after the adoption of the ICWA, Native American children continue to be overrepresented in foster care by a factor of two (Annie E. Casey Foundation 2019; U.S. Children's Bureau 2019).

TABLE 6–2. Summary of select federal child welfare legislation

Federal child welfare law	Purpose
Child Abuse Prevention and Treatment Act of 1974, Pub. L. 93-247, 88 Stat. 4 (1974) (CAPTA)	CAPTA provided grants to states for the purpose of preventing, identifying, and treating child abuse and neglect, defined by the act as "the physical or mental injury, sexual abuse, negligent treatment, or maltreatment of a child under the age of eighteen by a person who is responsible for the child's welfare under circumstances which indicate that the child's health or welfare is harmed or threatened thereby."
Indian Child Welfare Act of 1978, Pub. L. No. 95-608, 92 Stat. 3069 (ICWA)	ICWA was enacted to protect the best interests of Indian children and to promote stability of Indian tribes and families by establishing minimum standards for removal of an Indian child from his or her family and placement in foster care. The act created exclusive tribal jurisdiction over all Indian child custody proceedings—including child dependency, termination of parental rights, and adoption—when requested by the Tribe, parent, or Indian custodian and requires that Indian children be placed in foster or adoptive homes that reflect Indian culture.
Adoption Assistance and Child Welfare Act of 1980, Pub. L. 96-272 (AACWA)	AACWA was passed to decrease the need for out-of-home placement for children by requiring state child welfare agencies to make "reasonable efforts" to prevent removal, and when children are removed, to make "reasonable efforts" to reunify the family. The act also established federal funding to support state foster care and adoption assistance programs.
Multi-Ethnic Placement Act of 1994, Pub. L. No. 103-382, 108 Stat. 3518 (MEPA)	MEPA attempted to address issues of racial overrepresentation in the foster care system by prohibiting federally funded foster care and adoption agencies from delaying or denying a placement on the basis of the race or national origin of the child or the foster or adoptive parent.
Interethnic Placement provisions of 1996, Pub. L. No. 104-188, 110 Stat. 1755 (IEP)	IEP prohibited the use of race as a factor in placement decisions altogether.

TABLE 6–2.   Summary of select federal child welfare legislation *(continued)*

Federal child welfare law	Purpose
Adoption and Safe Families Act of 1997, Pub. L. 105-89 (ASFA)	ASFA affirmed child safety as the paramount concern of the child welfare system and stressed timely decision making for children and families. Its express aim is "to promote the adoption of children in foster care." The act authorized expedited permanency processes and permitted courts to excuse the agency from making "reasonable efforts" to reunify under certain circumstances. It also imposed strict time limits for moving a child to legal permanency, preferably through adoption.
Fostering Connections to Success and Increasing Adoptions Act of 2008, Pub. L. No. 110-351, 122 Stat. 3949 (FCSIAA)	FCSIAA mandated child welfare agencies to address certain domains of a child's well-being, including practices and procedures to identify and engage relatives, maintain sibling placements or visitation, undertake transition planning for older youth, ensure educational stability, and provide for ongoing oversight and coordination of health care needs and services.
Child and Family Services Improvement and Innovation Act of 2011, Pub. L. No. 112-34, 125 Stat. 369 (CFSIIA)	CFSIIA required states to develop a plan for oversight and coordination of health care services for children in foster care, including features addressing how emotional trauma would be monitored and treated and how psychotropic medications would be appropriately used and monitored. The act also emphasized the developmental needs of children in foster care, particularly those younger than age 5, and revised requirements for time-limited family reunification services to add peer-to-peer mentoring and support groups for parents and primary caregivers and services and activities to facilitate visitation between children in foster care and their parents and siblings.

For its part, the Adoption Assistance and Child Welfare Act of 1980 (AACWA) restored the emphasis of federal policy to a focus on family preservation in an attempt to prevent the unnecessary removal of children and placement in foster care. Simultaneously, however, AACWA created a separate entitlement funding stream to reimburse states for their foster care expenses while prevention and family reunification funding remained fixed. Thus, the financing of the system was discordant with its policy aims and strategies. The foster care system witnessed a near doubling as a result, as well as no improvement in children's length of stay in care (Roberts 2002).

The pendulum of child welfare policy soon swung in the other direction as high-profile accounts of child fatalities and serious injuries inflicted by parents triggered the instinct to separate families—in order to protect children (Roberts 1999). At the same time, the use of foster care was also drawing criticism, particularly concerning increasing lengths of stay and the overrepresentation of Black children (Roberts 1999). Congress reacted with the passage of new laws that accommodated, rather than challenged, the entrenched norms of the past. With its policy focus on *permanency*—the legal and emotional status of a child within a family—the Adoption and Safe Families Act of 1997 (ASFA) swung the policy pendulum decisively in the direction of child protection. Most notably, ASFA requires the state to file a petition to terminate parental rights when a child has been in foster care for 15 of the most recent 22 months. In the context that favors the archetypal family and a child-rescue philosophy, ASFA's policy and statutory mechanisms have not altered the trajectory for Black and Native American children. Twenty-two percent of the more than 125,000 children currently waiting to be adopted are Black, and 2% are Native American (U.S. Children's Bureau 2019). These statistics also offer a reflection on the success of the Multi-Ethnic Placement Act of 1994 (MEPA) and the Interethnic Placement provisions of 1996 (IEP) that amended MEPA. Together, these laws were meant to reduce barriers to permanency for children of color in foster care. The result of the passage of MEPA and IEP, however, was not racial equity but rather federal policy that favored transracial adoption, particularly the adoption of Black children in foster care, by white middle-class families, harkening back to the Native American assimilation argument (Roberts 2002).

With safety and permanency established as child welfare system outcomes and policy priorities, Congress next turned its attention to child well-being. A decade after ASFA, Congress passed the Fostering Connections to Success and Increasing Adoptions Act of 2008 (FCSIAA), which, among other policy reforms, requires state child welfare agencies to develop health care coordination and oversight plans for children in foster care in consultation with pediatricians and other health care experts. Such plans must specifically address mental health and dental services and the oversight of prescription medications, among other services. This focus was reinforced with the passage of the Child and Family Services Improvement and Innovation Act of 2011, which requires states to address the emotional trauma associated with maltreatment and removal and to describe how the use of psychotropic medications is monitored. With a focus on trauma and mental health treatment, these and other laws endeavor to elaborate on the meaning of the state's duty to ensure the welfare and well-being of children through specific directives regarding their care. None yet, however, have remedied the structural inequities of the system that undermine that very goal.

Mental Health and Child Welfare

The role of the mental health system in relation to the child welfare system cannot be explicated without the historical and institutional context of either system. In some ways, mental health needs serve as proxies for unaddressed social needs of marginalized families that have experienced discrimination and often lived in poverty for generations. Foster care placement instability is one area that reveals system-level contradictions to what is known to be in the best interest of children's healthy development. For children in foster care for more than 24 months, only 35% have fewer than two foster care placements; moreover, an increasing number of placements has been associated with a lower likelihood of reunification (Annie E. Casey Foundation 2018). Only 40% of states report that they have been able to achieve a goal of limiting the number of placements to two (Annie E. Casey Foundation 2018). Placement instability results in limited opportunities for children to feel safe in their home environment, connect with a caring adult, and establish competency in other areas, such as school or other activities. A change in placement may also mean a change in mental health providers. Although behavioral issues are often cited as the impetus for placement change, the variable preparation of foster parents, impact of the change in living environment, and turnover of caseworkers are institutional failures that factor into an unstable world that children are left to navigate.

Mental health professionals are often placed in a role in which they are asked to treat a child despite having limited information and limited contact with the family. Additionally, treatment of children is ineffective without knowledge of the aforementioned tension and deficiencies within the child welfare system. Mental health services are most often provided by mental health professionals outside the child welfare system and funded by Medicaid, for which children become eligible when they enter foster care. Because of the changes in insurance coverage, family instability, and sometimes multiple placements, treatment can be fractured, which contributes to poor treatment outcomes and engagement fatigue. Ironically, the cornerstone of therapy for maltreatment—establishing safety and predictability—is often undermined by both the child welfare system and the foster care system because of contractual changes, provider turnover, and limited engagement of biological families, leaving children continuously grappling with change and instability.

As the child welfare system and mental health system interact, the inequities in one naturally appear in the other, particularly when laws require and reinforce collaborations across systems. Mental health services are less likely to be provided to Black children and children within kinship care; in contrast, younger children with behavioral health concerns, children with more severe symptoms, and children in out-of-home placement are more likely to be seen by a mental health provider (Burns et al. 2004). Particularly for poor Black families in urban areas in which child welfare involvement may be prevalent, affiliated mental health services may be seen as coercive. Additionally, engaging in both systems can be stigmatizing on multiple levels. These inequities in treatment mirror the lower engagement of Black youth in mental health treatment among those not involved in the child welfare system. This lower engagement has been attributed to stigma, lack of culturally informed services, and the funneling of children with behavior problems into the juvenile justice system (Alegría et al. 2010), but it can also be understood as a function of decreased access to culturally informed or high-quality care in minority communities.

Promotion of trauma-informed, family-centered approaches should be the first line of intervention for many families; however, these services are often not widely disseminated and require a time course of dedicated treatment. A course can be compromised by lack of treatment coverage by Medicaid or loss of coverage due to change in placement or reunification. Ideally, these interventions would be preventive by design, with the engagement of families experiencing multiple stressors before the point at which child welfare involvement is even considered. Most commonly, however, service needs are identified after involvement with child welfare. Wraparound services, including home visits, parent support, and accessible psychotherapy, can be helpful to families facing multiple stressors (Garcia et al. 2013). Engagement in mental health services for children and families involved in the child welfare system is largely dependent on the identification of symptoms and knowledge of available and appropriate services. Once these issues are identified, the child welfare team, including a case manager and social worker, make recommendations regarding treatment.

In some ways, demands for mental health services with limited availability of psychotherapeutic treatments lead to psychotropic prescribing practices characterized as "too many, too much, and too young" (Fernandes-Alcantara et al. 2017, p. 14). Compared with children who are not in foster care, children in foster care are more likely to be prescribed multiple psychotropic medications, be prescribed higher doses of medication, and have higher rates of prescriptions at 0–6 years of age (Fernandes-Alcantara et al. 2017). Although psychotherapeutic interventions are the mainstay of treatment for children who experience maltreatment, psychotropic medications are used in 21%–39% of children in foster care, compared with 10% of children in the general population (Crystal et al. 2016). Children within the child welfare system can be some of the most complicated to treat clinically because they may exhibit symptoms across the diagnostic spectrum due to experiences of trauma and chronic maltreatment. Unfortunately, children's mental health providers are asked to treat psychosocial ills of poverty, family disruption, and adverse childhood experiences with a limited toolkit within a system that is constrained by time, funding, and regulatory policies.

Future Directions for Child Welfare

The child welfare system is yet again poised for transformation, this time through a constellation of long-anticipated policies that create an opportunity to reorient the system's focus from intervention to prevention and, in doing so, to maintain families of origin. The recently enacted Family First Prevention Services Act (Family First Act), included in the Bipartisan Budget Act of 2018, is the most significant piece of federal child welfare legislation in decades, and it holds the potential to dramatically change the nation's child welfare system. Through refinancing of federal funding, state child welfare agencies will, for the first time, have access to an entitlement funding stream for prevention services. In this way, child welfare system funding will achieve the long-needed alignment with prevention and family preservation goals as robustly as it has been historically aligned with out-of-home placement. The primary policy aims of the Family First Act are 1) to prevent the unnecessary placement of children in foster care and 2) to promote family-based care for children who cannot remain safely at home. Although the law is not designed explicitly to address racial inequities, the aims of strengthening and supporting families are centrally responsive to the experience of Black and Indigenous children and families in the child welfare system.

Under the Family First Act, states will determine which children are at imminent risk of entering foster care, and those candidates—along with pregnant and parenting youth in foster care and the parents, kin caregivers, and nonrelative guardians of such children and youth—will be deemed eligible for evidence-based mental health, substance use treatment and prevention, and parenting skills services. The return to a clear emphasis on family preservation rather than removal is justified by the growing body of evidence pointing to interventions that are effective at addressing family problems that, left unaddressed, create risk for child maltreatment and the potential for family separation as the system responds.

Despite this new legal path to services, however, challenges of access to and availability of such evidence-based treatments remain throughout the mental health system for all children. Thus, as history has demonstrated, the promise of a new law reinforcing the policy of family preservation does not ensure equity in the receipt of services or outcomes. The goal of family preservation cannot be realized fully without confronting the history of structural racism and classism in the policies and practices of the child welfare system. A system designed to promote the prosperity of families and the well-being of children must acknowledge the roles that race and poverty play in the engagement of families in times of greatest need.

Questions for Self-Reflection

1. What do I know about the function of the child welfare system in my community?
2. In what ways might the child welfare system protect, neglect, or harm children?
3. What are my professional experiences with the child welfare system? In what ways might the "care" provided be helping or harming patients through these interactions?

References

Alegría M, Vallas M, Pumariega AJ: Racial and ethnic disparities in pediatric mental health. Child Adolesc Psychiatr Clin North Am 19:759–774, 2010

Annie E. Casey Foundation: What impacts placement stability? Strategy Brief: Strong Families, Seattle, WA, Casey Family Programs, October 3, 2018. Available at www.casey.org/placement-stability-impacts. Accessed April 19, 2020.

Annie E. Casey Foundation: Child population by race in the United States. Baltimore, MD, Kids Count Data Center, Annie E. Casey Foundation, August 2019. Available at: https://datacenter.kidscount.org/data/tables/103-child-population-by-race. Accessed May 10, 2020.

Billingsley A, Giovannoni JM: Children of the Storm: Black Children and American Child Welfare. New York, Harcourt Brace Jovanovich, 1972

Brice TS: Child welfare practice: an African-centered approach, J Hum Behav Soc Environ 27:81–91, 2017

Burns BJ, Phillips SD, Wagner HR, et al: Mental health need and access to mental health services by youths involved with child welfare: a national survey. J Am Acad Child Adolesc Psychiatry 43:960–970, 2004

Crystal S, Mackie T, Fenton MC, et al: Rapid growth of antipsychotic prescriptions for children who are publicly insured has ceased, but concerns remain. Health Aff 35:974–982, 2016

Ensign K: The Federal Role in Foster Care: A Paper on Current Priority Issue Areas. Washington, DC, U.S. Department of Health and Human Services, 1989

Fernandes-Alcantara AL, Caldwell SW, Stoltzfus E: Child Welfare: Oversight of Psychotropic Medication for Children in Foster Care. Congressional Research Service, 2017

Garcia AR, Palinkas LA, Snowden L, Landsverk J: Looking beneath and in between the hidden surfaces: a critical review of defining, measuring and contextualizing mental health service disparities in the child welfare system. Child Youth Serv Rev 35:1727–1733, 2013

Garcia AR, Circo E, DeNard C, Hernandez N: Barriers and facilitators to delivering effective mental health practice strategies for youth and families served by the child welfare system. Child Youth Serv Rev 52:110–122, 2015

Garland AF, Landsverk JL, Hough RL, Ellis-MacLeod E: Type of maltreatment as a predictor of mental health service use for children in foster care. Child Abuse Negl 20:675–688, 1996

Harris M: Racial Disproportionality in Child Welfare. New York, Columbia University Press, 2014

Hill RB: Institutional racism in child welfare. Race Soc 7:17–33, 2004

Hill RB: Disproportionality of Minorities in Child Welfare: Synthesis of Research Findings. Baltimore, MD, Annie E. Casey Foundation, 2006. Available at: https://pdfs.semanticscholar.org/bf24/537ccd20dc9b9807ff6c8e22c62d254 b6e00.pdf. Accessed May 8, 2020.

Holt MI: The Orphan Trains: Placing Out in America. Lincoln, NE, Bison Books, 1994

Jacobs MD: Remembering the "forgotten child": the American Indian child welfare crisis of the 1960s and 1970s. Am Indian Q 37:136–159, 2013

Jalongo MR: The story of Mary Ellen Wilson: tracing the origins of child protection in America. Early Child Educ J 34:1–4, 2006

Meyer v. Nebraska, 262 U.S. 390, 1923

Myers JEB: A short history of child protection in America. Fam Law Q 42:449–463, 2008

Pelton LH: Not for poverty alone: foster care population trends in the twentieth century. J Sociol Soc Welf 14:37–61, 1987

Pierce v. Society of Sisters, 268 U.S. 510, 1925

Prince v. Massachusetts, 321 U.S. 158, 1944

Roberts DE: Is there justice in children's rights: the critique of federal family preservation policy. Univ Pa J Const Law 2:112–140, 1999

Roberts DE: Shattered Bonds: The Color of Child Welfare. New York, Basic Civitas Books, 2002

Sedlak AJ, Mettenburg J, Basena M, et al: Fourth National Incidence Study of Child Abuse and Neglect (NIS-4): Report to Congress. Washington, DC, U.S. Department of Health and Human Services, 2010

Social Security Act of 1935, Pub. L. No. 74-271, 49 Stat. 620, 1935

Trammell RS: Orphan train myths and legal reality. Modern American 5:3–13, 2009

U.S. Children's Bureau: The Story of the White House Conferences on Children. Washington DC, Children's Bureau, 1967

U.S. Children's Bureau: Racial Disproportionality and Disparity in Child Welfare. Washington DC, Children's Bureau, November 2016. Available at www.childwelfare.gov/pubpdfs/racial_disproportionality.pdf. Accessed May 11, 2020.

U.S. Children's Bureau: The AFCARS Report. Washington DC, Children's Bureau, October 24, 2019. Available at www.acf.hhs.gov/sites/default/files/cb/afcarsreport26.pdf. Accessed May 3, 2020.

U.S. Children's Bureau: Child Maltreatment 2018. Washington DC, Children's Bureau, January 15, 2020. Available at www.acf.hhs.gov/cb/research-data-technology /statistics-research/child-maltreatment. Accessed May 3, 2020.

CHAPTER 7

Social Injustice and Urban Development

Jacob Michael Izenberg, M.D.
Mindy Thompson Fullilove, M.D.

The Saga of Detroit

Greektown is one the few preserved, pedestrian-friendly districts reminiscent of pre-World War II Detroit, Michigan. But walk just a few blocks east and you will encounter the Chrysler Freeway, one of the city's many expansive ribbons of multilane interstate, coursing through a vast man-made canyon (Figure 7–1). What you will not encounter are the neighborhoods of Black Bottom and Paradise Valley. These districts were once home to most of the city's Black residents; Black-owned businesses; and Black cultural institutions, such as the New Bethel Baptist Church, where Aretha Franklin first sang. The neighborhood's main thoroughfare, Hastings, once ran on level ground, where the concrete chasm now lies.

Historian Thomas Sugrue (1996) has detailed how early twentieth-century migrants from the Jim Crow South, unwelcome in most of Detroit's white neighborhoods, moved in large numbers to Black Bottom and Paradise Valley. There they created economically dynamic and culturally rich

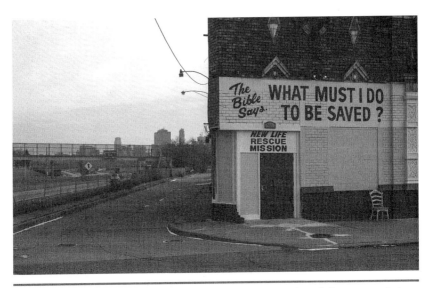

FIGURE 7–1. The Fisher Freeway, one example of the many interstates cutting through Detroit.
To view this figure in color, see Plate 2 in Color Gallery.

communities, even after often being forced to live in crowded and deteriorating buildings, restricted in their options and cut off from investment and financing. Despite the vibrancy of these neighborhoods, Detroit's white leaders designated them slums and, enabled by new federal programs in the postwar era, moved to dismantle them—piecemeal at first, with money from the American Housing Act of 1949, and then wholesale, through freeway construction (Sugrue 1996). Thus began the long decline of postwar Detroit through a series of wounds: flight to the suburbs by white residents, riots stemming from anger over racism and economic exclusion, abandonment by the auto industry and other manufacturers, cuts to the social safety net, the withdrawal of municipal services, and a foreclosure crisis—one rooted in exploitative lending practices—that decimated many Detroit families (Sugrue 1996).

In recent years, Detroit has laid claim to a comeback built on resurgent national interest in the dynamism of urban life. However, the experience of Detroit should warn us that the inequity that shaped the urban decline will also shape the renaissance, absent a broad effort toward a more inclusive alternative. So far, the city's power brokers and newcomers, many of them white, have been disproportionate beneficiaries of the New Detroit (Williams 2020).

Detroit's story, while perhaps noteworthy in its scale, nevertheless captures principles of urban injustice that are common to many American cities. First, our cities are *sorted out*—segregated by race, first and foremost, as well as by class (Fullilove 2013). Second, poor neighborhoods—and in particular those of color—have been repeatedly targeted for disinvestment, dismantling, and displacement, all of which are processes that have undermined community stability and produced repetitive collective trauma. Third, because of the American consensus that housing is a commodity rather than a right, unaffordability, instability, and housing-related economic exploitation are common, compounding inequity. These processes have collectively helped establish a racialized geography of social injustice in major American cities: wealthier neighborhoods, many of them predominantly white, get a surplus of opportunity, advantages, and abundant resources, whereas poorer neighborhoods, particularly those of color, have an overrepresentation of noxious environmental features, economic marginalization, and social problems.

Our central task in this chapter is to link this situation to mental health. We begin by reviewing in more detail some of the history that has gotten us here and then turn to the collective social dynamics of urban neighborhoods as a reemerging explanatory link to community mental health and well-being. We wrote this chapter with the hope that efforts guided by a deeper understanding of the psychological impact of the sorted-out city—whether they be in research, policy making, program development, clinical care, or community building and citizenship—will be better equipped to yield a more just urban environment for mental health.

The Legacy of Injustice in Twentieth-Century Urban Policy

Segregation

The American city is segregated by race and, perhaps to a lesser extent, class. In fact, segregation is such a pervasive fact of urban life in the United States that it might be hard to picture things otherwise, yet, prior to the turn of the twentieth century, American cities were generally less segregated than they are today (Shertzer and Walsh 2019). The urban historian Thomas Hanchett (1998), in describing the process by which American cities got sorted out, characterized post-Reconstruction-era Charlotte, North Carolina neighborhoods as "salt-and-pepper," which is to say that white and Black households were interspersed among one another. In contrast to the South, Northern cities at the end of the Civil War still had relatively few Black residents. That began to change as Black Southerners, seeking refuge from racial violence and economic exclusion, moved in large numbers to newly industrializing urban centers in the North and West (Tolnay 2003). Known as the *Great Migration*, this movement gave rise to Northern cities' first significant Black populations and, as recent statistical analysis has suggested, to an early version of a pattern that was repeated often in later decades, whereby white Northerners moved to more racially homogeneous neighborhoods as Black residents settled nearby (Shertzer and Walsh 2019). Meanwhile, by the mid-twentieth century, Charlotte, like many other Southern cities, had become a checkerboard of racially homogeneous neighborhoods (Hanchett 1998).

Twentieth-century urban segregation was not simply an individual choice in aggregate or the happenstance of socioeconomics; as Rothstein (2017) detailed in great depth, it was frequently de jure, a matter of law. In 1916, New York City introduced the first citywide ordinance for *comprehensive zoning*, whereby the government could place parameters on private land use (Platt 2014). Growing in part from a desire to insulate residential areas from industrial land uses and otherwise help shape the unruly growth of cities in the early twentieth century, zoning also has roots in racial exclusion. Indeed, nearly a decade before New York's zoning law, the city of Baltimore, Maryland, enacted a law prohibiting the movement of Black residents into white neighborhoods, and vice versa (Silver 1991). Until they were ruled unconstitutional by the Supreme Court's *Buchannan v. Warley* (1917) ruling, these types of explicitly segregationist zoning ordinances proliferated (Rothstein 2017). Even after *Buchannan*, well into the 1920s, cities made efforts to skirt the ruling by tweaking their ordinances on the margins; these efforts were often defeated in court, but not before cities had collectively exerted several decades' worth of discriminatory pressure (Silver 1991).

Throughout the same era, another widely used tool of segregation was the *restrictive covenant*, in which a property deed would mandate that owners could sell only to white buyers or rent only to white tenants. It was not until *Shelley v. Kraemer* (1948), some 30 years after *Buchannan*, that the Supreme Court ruled such covenants unenforceable. Subsequently, individuals who were intent on racial apartheid deployed other types of exclusionary zoning such as density limits, which, in combination with other practices limiting Blacks' and other minority groups' access to single-family housing, continue to perpetuate racial segregation to this day (Rothstein 2017).

As neighborhood segregation was often promoted and enforced through law, so too was the segregation of public housing. From the New Deal era through the 1970s, the federal government subsidized the construction of millions of public housing units (Schwartz 2014). The first significant federal housing legislation, the U.S. Housing Act of 1937, devolved to local public housing authorities responsibility for overseeing most aspects of public housing, including where and whether to build these units (von Hoffman 1996). The extensive authority afforded to local governments encouraged segregation, allowing city governments to preferentially concentrate housing projects in Black neighborhoods or designate housing projects in white neighborhoods (while it was still legal to do so) for white tenants only (Schwartz 2014). Frequently, white communities simply refused to build any public housing at all (Rothstein 2017).

The federal government also promoted residential segregation by enforcing policies that gave whites preferential access to homeownership. Rothstein (2017) has detailed the instruments involved in this process. These include the Home Owners' Loan Corporation (HOLC), which purchased bad Depression-era mortgages from private banks in order to refinance them, as well as the Federal Housing Administration (FHA) and the Veterans Administration (VA), which provided backing for countless home mortgages and helped finance millions of new units of housing (Rothstein 2017). HOLC was short-lived, but it earned outsized notoriety for effectively inventing *redlining*, the practice of creating color-coded neighborhood investment-worthiness maps, giving poor grades (red) to neighborhoods with residents of color. The FHA and VA were major players in the housing market, and for several decades they required segregation as a condition of financing (Rothstein 2017), spurring developers to go to remarkable lengths in dividing Black and white urban neighborhoods. In one infamous case, a developer in Detroit built a wall separating a new all-white neighborhood from a neighboring Black community in order to secure financing (Kozlowski 2019). Racism in federal lending not only provided white families with a major economic advantage, but also, by preferentially encouraging their ability to move to suburbs, effectively supercharged so-called *white flight* from urban neighborhoods.

The Supreme Court's *Brown v. Board of Education* (1954) decision legally ended the practice of racial segregation, at least in principle. Major civil rights laws during the President Lyndon Johnson era codified many of the tenets of equal justice under the law, answering a grassroots movement with federal legislation protecting people of color from discrimination. These acts represented significant progress toward racial justice and have been rightly celebrated. However, none of them actually ended racism in urban policy and housing (or in voting, law enforcement, or any other domain of public life). Nor did they undo a prior half-century of segregation and stratification in urban neighborhoods. By the end of the 1960s (a decade that contained both the promise of federal civil rights action and the reality of urban renewal), racist backlash, major urban riots, and the acceleration of white flight out of American cities ensured that urban racial segregation remained as serious and pervasive as it had ever been.

Redlining, Disinvestment, and the Repeated Dismantling of Neighborhoods of Color

Detroit planners were able to route the Chrysler Freeway through a Black neighborhood because there *was* a Black neighborhood. In a sorted-out city, policies targeting people of color can be veiled—thin though the veil may be—by other prerogatives of government. Redlining, disinvestment, urban renewal, selective placement of toxic and polluting land uses, planned shrinkage, overpolicing and mass incarceration, economic exploitation, and policies promoting gentrification all leverage the divided city to target Black neighborhoods while publicly claiming to serve other purposes—slum clearance, preservation of land values, efficiency of city services, reduction of crime, bolstering of development, and so forth. We will turn our attention now to some of these processes and the enormous impact they have had.

Although it has become a catch-all for describing many phenomena related to residential segregation, *redlining* as a concept is arguably more useful in understanding what has happened to particular neighborhoods during the mid-twentieth century, as opposed to what gave rise to them in earlier decades. As described in the previous subsection, redlining refers to the color-coded residential security maps created by HOLC during the Great Depression to help guide residential lending and mortgage support. Neighborhood racial makeup was a key part of these assessments; those areas in which racial minority groups were represented received the *high-risk* designation and were shaded red on a map (Figure 7–2). This designation promoted the degradation of these neighborhoods by discouraging the financing of home ownership and building improvements (Rothstein 2017). Cut off from such investment, many redlined areas saw their building stock in significant physical decline by the end of the Depression era.

The Housing Act of 1949 introduced the program that came to be known as *urban renewal*, which allocated federal funds for *slum clearance* efforts and, ostensibly, replacement with new housing. Urban renewal grew in part out of the claim by progressive supporters of environmental determinism that the deteriorating physical conditions of many inner-city neighborhoods were themselves responsible for various health and social problems of urban life (von Hoffman 2010). Many city governments, however, saw in urban renewal the opportunity to disperse minority neighborhoods in order to reclaim them for other uses. Indeed, so transparently did urban renewal tend to target neighborhoods of color that among many activists it earned the moniker *Negro removal* (Fullilove 2005; Rothstein 2017; Sugrue 1996).

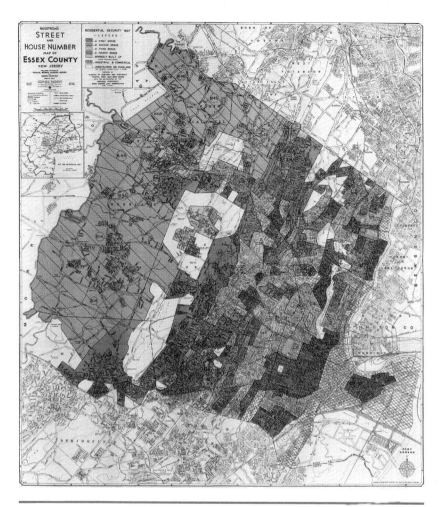

FIGURE 7–2. Residential security map of Essex County, New Jersey, produced in 1939.
To view this figure in color, see Plate 3 in Color Gallery.
Source. Courtesy of the National Archives, Washington, DC.

Cities, rather than rebuilding the housing that was lost, often created commercial developments, civic centers and arenas, or interstates, all of which served the commercial interests of the predominantly white middle and upper classes (Teaford 2010). The minority neighborhoods that survived urban renewal and highway construction found themselves riven by swaths of pavement or severed from the urban core by these massive developments and driven further into decline as a result (Fullilove 2005). Also, although they came at great human cost, many of the developments created by urban planning were devoid of the vitality that defined the neighborhoods they replaced, coming before long to be seen as failures (Jacobs 1961).

Where did the displaced residents of these neighborhoods wind up? In many cases, they occupied the massive high-rise public housing projects built as part of the urban renewal effort itself. These towers were often purposefully built to be cut off from other areas of the city, isolating their residents. Because they were overwhelmingly occupied by low-income families, rents were not sufficient to pay for maintenance, which allowed the properties to rapidly deteriorate (Schwartz 2014). In other cases, those individuals displaced by urban renewal moved into adjacent neighborhoods abandoned by white flight, where cycles of disinvestment, decline, and displacement were in many cases repeated. Wherever they ultimately ended up, individuals displaced by urban renewal found their communities dismantled and alienated, the ties that once bound people together strained and broken under the weight of the scattering (Fullilove and Wallace 2011).

Urban deindustrialization in the 1970s compounded the economic distress of inner-city neighborhoods of color as steady manufacturing and industrial jobs left urban centers (Wilson 1991). Cuts to federal housing and welfare programs in the 1980s and 1990s dismantled much of what passed for an economic and social safety net. *Planned shrinkage*, the deliberate withdrawal of city services from struggling neighborhoods, allowed targeted areas to deteriorate further and, in particular, left them vulnerable to the ravages of fire—as was seen so vividly when much of New York City's Bronx burned throughout the 1970s (Wallace 1993). The "War on Drugs" compounded overpolicing and mass incarceration, particularly of Black men (Cooper and Fullilove 2020; Fullilove and Wallace 2011). Each of these issues has been the subject of a great deal of scholarly attention. Their brief mention here is meant to serve the point that once residential segregation and redlining practices had been established, the stage was set for the repetitive assaults on neighborhoods of color.

The processes described above have left the very same neighborhoods open to economic exploitation, sometimes termed *reverse redlining*. Such practices, in fact, go back well into the twentieth century, when landlords would often levy excessive rents on Black tenants, knowing they had few other options, and real estate speculators would engage in *blockbusting*—inflaming racial fears to deflate the sale prices of white-owned homes before reselling them to Black buyers at inflated prices (Rothstein 2017). Today, economic exploitation is a major problem in poor neighborhoods, regardless of race, although it continues to disproportionately affect people of color. Excessive rent burdens continue to be common in Black neighborhoods, leading to regular displacement and instability in the form of eviction. This problem is so widespread that sociologist Matthew Desmond

(2012) has argued that "in poor black neighborhoods, eviction is to women what incarceration is to men: a typical but severely consequential occurrence contributing to the reproduction of urban poverty" (p. 88). Subprime lending has also disproportionately targeted neighborhoods of color, as was seen to devastating effect during the 2008 Great Recession, when families of color lost, on average, a far larger percentage of their wealth than did white families (Desmond 2016).

As with Detroit, many cities are seeing renewed middle- and upper-class interest in urban living. Perhaps more importantly, developers and speculators have started to once again view the city as a good place to invest, particularly in previously disinvested neighborhoods, which are often located close to city centers (Lees et al. 2008). Bringing the specter of rapid community change and rising costs of living, gentrification poses a new potential for destabilization and displacement in neighborhoods of color. Even without physical displacement, the rapid changes happening in these neighborhoods risk alienation and community disruption, as evidenced by the frequently acrimonious debates—often deeply informed by experiences of past racial injustice—that have arisen in many of the neighborhoods facing significant gentrification.

Thus far, we have detailed several key points in a troubling history of social injustice in American cities. In the end, this history is not just about the result: unequal, sorted-out cities. It is also about *how* we got here, through what might best be described as chronic neglect and repetitive trauma. In individual people, these conditions often produce syndromes such as PTSD. What about for the city and its inhabitants?

Mental Health in the Social Context

Collective Efficacy and Well-Being

In 1897, sociologist Emile Durkheim described a particular type of suicide he had observed in which individuals were responding to a breakdown in the social integration necessary for human thriving, a condition he referred to as *anomie* (Berkman et al. 2000). The long-term Stirling County Study, which sought in the mid-twentieth century to examine the prevalence and correlates of mental illness in a region of Nova Scotia, found that those communities with higher levels of social integration had lower rates of psychiatric distress when compared with those with less social integration (Leighton et al. 1963). Stemming from observations such as these, the idea that community social integration is important for mental (and physical) health has remained a guiding principle for social psychiatrists and psychologists, while slowly gaining broader acceptance in the public health community (Berkman et al. 2000).

This makes sense. Humans are, after all, social beings—participation in communities is an essential feature of human life, something we are, in effect, wired for. Community dynamics have the potential to affect members through a complex array of pathways operating at multiple levels, including the direct psychological and physiological impact of social intimacy and support, access to material goods and opportunity, the regulation of behavior, the achievement of collective goals, resistance to structural violence, and resilience in the face of trauma or disaster (Berkman et al. 2000). We are so closely bound to these contexts that, as Nancy Krieger (2012) has put it, we come to literally *embody* them.

Sociologist Robert Sampson (1997), in an effort to more precisely characterize the community-level dynamics that might influence rates of violent crime, described *collective efficacy*, a community's capacity to act collectively on shared norms and values, regulate social behavior, and achieve mutual objectives. The concept of collective efficacy is useful because it is more precisely defined than some other commonly used terms describing social cohesion, such as *social capital*, and because it directly addresses how communities *function*, such as through collective action, standards of public participation, and behavioral norms. This principle can be seen in operation in the neighborhoods of Chicago, Illinois, where individuals with higher collective efficacy "seem to do better on a lot of...things [in addition to lower crime rates], including birth weight, rates of teen pregnancy, and infant mortality, suggesting a link to overall health and well-being independent of social composition. *In most cases, then, whether rich or poor, white or black, I argue that collective efficacy signals a community on a trajectory of well-being*" (Sampson 2012, p. 368).

In recent years, a growing body of research has substantiated this thesis. Among adolescents, for example, high community collective efficacy is linked to reduced rates of anxiety and depression (Donnelly et al. 2017), high-risk sexual behavior (Browning et al. 2008), and substance use (Vaeth et al. 2015). Among adults, high collective efficacy has been linked to lower rates of major depression (Ahern and Galea 2011). Neighborhoods with higher collective efficacy tend to have lower rates of violent crime (Sampson 1997). In this era of the growing climate crisis, when weather-related disasters may become increasingly common, it is noteworthy that recent research on Florida communities affected by major hurricanes found that, controlling for the degree of exposure to trauma, those living in areas with higher collective efficacy were less likely to experience PTSD (Fullerton et al. 2019).

As stated earlier, Sampson (2012) noted the importance of collective efficacy in neighborhoods, "whether rich or poor," suggesting that perhaps collective efficacy is as important as (or perhaps even more important than) socioeconomic status when it comes to matters of community well-being. This is an idea worth investigating further. Another striking finding of the Stirling County Study offers some insight: in the more socially cohesive communities studied, even individuals at the lowest end of the socioeconomic spectrum were at lower risk for psychiatric symptoms than were those at the upper end of disintegrated communities (Leighton et al. 1963). More recent research has corroborated the idea that at the neighborhood level, collective efficacy may be a more reliable predictor of well-being than socioeconomic disadvantage. For example, Browning and Cagney (2002) found that when controlling for individual-level factors, neighborhood collective efficacy—but not neighborhood socioeconomic status—was correlated with self-rated health (a broad indicator that not only is tied to mental well-being but also is correlated with objective measures of health, such as mortality). Later work has supported this research, suggesting that low collective efficacy may be a key mediator for the effect of concentrated disadvantage on overall health and on mental health specifically (Cohen et al. 2003; Xue et al. 2005). Taken in aggregate, these findings suggest that, although the importance of neighborhood economic conditions should not be discounted, the social conditions of the neighborhood may have as much or more to tell us about mental health.

Collective Trauma and Community Breakdown

In the 1990s, ecologist Rodrick Wallace argued that the "loss of social control,...failure to properly socialize adolescents, intensification of individual anomie and...loss of community coping mechanisms for ameliorating such anomie" helped propel the spread of HIV/AIDS in a Bronx community devastated by the withdrawal of municipal services and the widespread fires and community displacement that resulted (Wallace 1993, p. 888). Although his work predated the term *collective efficacy*, Wallace was, in effect, describing the same thing, and in doing so provided a road map for better understanding how the injustices of urban policy might ultimately lead to illness.

The concept of collective efficacy was developed to address the observation that the density of close social ties may not be sufficient to explain outcomes often attributed to *social disorganization*, given that neighborhoods often deemed to be suffering such a state are in fact home to many close-knit networks of family and friends (Sampson 2012). What *is* missing, then?

Sampson (2012) argued that the answer lies in so-called *weak ties*, the social connections linking not family and friends but rather more loosely affiliated people from different groups—thereby bridging the gaps between them. Weak ties yield the community-wide information sharing and trust that are foundational to collective efficacy (Sampson 2012). According to this reasoning, when these ties are broken, collective efficacy is diminished.

And why might they be broken? We return to the sorted-out city. Fullilove and Wallace (2011), in reviewing the history of what they termed the *serial forced displacement* of minority communities in American cities, observed the evolution of social life in the Hill District of Pittsburgh, Pennsylvania. An area into which Black migrants were segregated, the Hill District was subjected (not without active resistance from many community members, it should be noted) to the range of policies described earlier in this chapter: redlining, disinvestment, urban renewal, and massive displacement; isolation from downtown by those same developments; deindustrialization; and further disinvestment from a deeply stressed urban fabric. One of the primary effects of these repeated assaults on the community fabric was the progressive diminishment of the neighborhood's social organization: whereas it had once been a "strong community composed of many organizations" (p. 385) with political strength and a "net of relationships that anchored the young" (p. 386), by the end of the twentieth century, the community had devolved to a patchwork of family units struggling against isolation and deep uncertainty (Fullilove and Wallace 2011). According to the logic of the Hill District's transformation, a plausible narrative linking the injustices of America's urban system to mental health can be traced through the history of the repetitive traumas visited on neighborhoods of color and their impact on collective efficacy.

Time and again, students of cities have observed the social and physical disruption of communities, brought about in a fashion like that seen in Pittsburgh and Detroit. The impact of sorting, disinvestment, and mass displacement was devastating in cities across the country, where the effects have continued to propagate through the urban space as new fronts of displacement have sprung from older ones. Examples of these other fronts, described briefly in an earlier section, include deindustrialization, which undercuts stable economic opportunity in urban neighborhoods (Wilson 1991); planned shrinkage, which has led to widespread destruction of housing by fire and widespread community breakdown (Wallace 1993); economic exploitation and eviction, which deeply destabilize the lives of poor Americans and undermine the social organization and resources of affected communities (Desmond 2018); and gentrification, which threatens displacement and exclusion (Lees et al. 2008). These successive waves of community destabilization and destruction are imprinted on the urban fabric itself: in some communities, Main

Streets are no longer "hospitable" to routine social engagement in the public space, a type of interaction that may be necessary for sustaining weak ties and, thus, collective efficacy (Izenberg and Fullilove 2016).

Healing the Whole City

Thanks to the discriminatory machinery by which urban neighborhoods have been undermined in the twentieth century, American cities are defined by deep and durable spatial inequality along lines of race, as well as class—not only in socioeconomic status but also in the quality and strength of collective efficacy (Sampson 2012). This situation and the repeated traumas by which we arrived at it pose significant mental health risks for the those residing in (and displaced from) the communities scarred by this structural violence. But the risks are not only for them. As grows the scale of our collective problems— regional housing crises and global climate change being examples—so grows the scale of collective action needed to solve them. Yet, driven by the social strain of sorting and inequality (Pickett and Wilkinson 2010), we seem divided just as we need to come together. As is often the case with injustice, there are no winners: although some people on top may seem to be winning, in the long run, the destruction of community sets up a reckoning.

There is no shortage of policy ideas that might begin to heal the wounds of sorting and displacement. Structural approaches might include reform of zoning codes to promote inclusion in more communities, adequate funding of transit systems that connect people, increased investment in affordable housing programs, and redress of the increasingly profound economic inequality that inevitably reflects itself in divided urban space. Programmatic responses, such as investment and development approaches that respect communities' rights, needs, and aspirations, might also be deployed. Architectural responses would include projects to repair and sustain beloved urban places, rather than destroy them, or to create landscapes and public spaces that reconnect neighborhoods divided by highways and other rifts in the urban fabric. Finally, social responses could include efforts to support grassroots community exchange and connection. Maybe what is most important is simply letting cities teach us. As the urbanist Jane Jacobs (1961) observed, "Vital cities have marvelous innate abilities for understanding, communicating, contriving, and inventing what is required to combat their difficulties" (p. 447). If we can start by acknowledging the structural violence that has occurred there, our sorted-out cities—capable as they are of fostering vibrant community life, grassroots organization, massive social and political change, scientific advancement, and artistic creativity, just to name a few of their achievements—might also offer us a path to healing.

Questions for Self-Reflection

1. What choices and priorities went into the decision I made about where I live? How have these decisions impacted my life? For my patients, what choices and priorities go into the decisions about where they live?
2. What do I know about the impact of redlining and residential segregation in the neighborhoods where I live and work?
3. How might urban development policies influence the social determinants of mental health in my patients?

References

Ahern J, Galea S: Collective efficacy and major depression in urban neighborhoods. Am J Epidemiol 173:1453–1462, 2011

Berkman L, Glass T, Brissette I, Seeman T: From social integration to health: Durkheim in the new millennium. Soc Sci Med 51:843–857, 2000

Brown v. Board of Education of Topeka, 347 U.S. 483, 1954

Browning CR, Cagney KA: Neighborhood structural disadvantage, collective efficacy, and self-rated physical health in an urban setting. J Health Soc Behav 43:383–399, 2002

Browning CR, Burrington LA, Leventhal T, Brooks-Gunn J: Neighborhood structural inequality, collective efficacy, and sexual risk behavior among urban youth. J Health Soc Behav 49:269–285, 2008

Buchannan v. Warley, 245 U.S. 60, 1917

Cohen DA, Farley TA, Mason K: Why is poverty unhealthy? Social and physical mediators. Soc Sci Med 57:1631–1641, 2003

Cooper HLF, Fullilove MT: From Enforcers to Guardians: A Public Health Primer on Ending Police Violence. Baltimore, MD, Johns Hopkins University Press, 2020

Desmond M: Eviction and the reproduction of urban poverty. Am J Sociol 118:88–133, 2012

Desmond M: Evicted. New York, Crown Publishing, 2016

Desmond M: Heavy is the house: rent burden among the American urban poor. Int J Urban Reg Res 42:160–170, 2018

Donnelly L, McLanahan S, Brooks-Gunn J, et al: Cohesive neighborhoods where social expectations are shared may have positive impact on adolescent mental health. Health Aff 35:2083–2091, 2017

Fullerton CS, Mash HB, Wang L, et al: Posttraumatic stress disorder and mental distress following the 2004 and 2005 Florida hurricanes. Disaster Med Public Health Prep 13:44–52, 2019

Fullilove MT: Root Shock. New York, Random House, 2005

Fullilove MT: Urban Alchemy. New York, New Village Press, 2013

Fullilove MT, Wallace R: Serial forced displacement in American cities, 1916–2010. J Urban Health 88:381–389, 2011

Hanchett T: Sorting out the New South City. Chapel Hill, University of North Carolina Press, 1998

Izenberg JM, Fullilove MT: Hospitality invites sociability, which builds cohesion: a model for the role of main streets in population mental health. J Urban Health 93:292–311, 2016

Jacobs J: The Death and Life of Great American Cities. New York, Vintage, 1961

Kozlowski K: Wall built to separate whites, blacks in Detroit "an important story to tell." Detroit News, July 9, 2019

Krieger N: Methods for the scientific study of discrimination and health: an ecosocial approach. Am J Public Health 102:936–944, 2012

Lees L, Slater T, Wyly E: Gentrification. New York, Taylor and Francis, 2008

Leighton DC, Harding JS, Macklin DB, et al: Psychiatric findings of the Stirling County study. Am J Psychiatry 119:1021–1026, 1963

Pickett KE, Wilkinson RG: Inequality: an underacknowledged source of mental illness and distress. Br J Psychiatry 197:426–428, 2010

Platt RH: Land Use and Society, 3rd Edition. Washington, DC, Island Press, 2014

Rothstein R: The Color of Law. New York, Liveright, 2017

Sampson RJ: Neighborhoods and violent crime: a multilevel study of collective efficacy. Science 277:918–924, 1997

Sampson RJ: Great American City: Chicago and the Enduring Neighborhood Effect. Chicago, IL, University of Chicago Press, 2012

Schwartz AF: Housing Policy in the United States, 3rd Edition. New York, Taylor and Francis, 2014

Shelley v. Kraemer, 334 U.S. 1, 1948

Shertzer A, Walsh RP: Racial sorting and the emergence of segregation in American cities. Rev Econ Stat 101:415–427, 2019

Silver C: The racial origins of zoning: Southern cities from 1910–40. Plan Perspect 6:189–205, 1991

Sugrue TJ: The Origins of the Urban Crisis: Race and Inequality in Post War Detroit. Princeton, NJ, Princeton University Press, 1996

Teaford JC: Urban renewal and its aftermath. Hous Policy Debate 11:443–465, 2010

Tolnay SE: The African American 'Great Migration' and beyond. Annu Rev Sociol 29:209–232, 2003

Vaeth PA, Caetano R, Mills BA: Binge drinking and perceived neighborhood characteristics among Mexican Americans residing on the U.S.-Mexico border. Alcohol Clin Exp Res 39:1727–1733, 2015

von Hoffman A: High ambitions: the past and future of American low-income housing policy. Hous Policy Debate 7:423–446, 1996

von Hoffman A: A study in contradictions: the origins and legacy of the Housing Act of 1949. Hous Policy Debate 11:299–326, 2010

Wallace R: Social disintegration and the spread of AIDS. Soc Sci Med 37:887–896, 1993

Williams J: A Tale of Two Motor Cities: as the city climbs out of decades of decline, many of Detroit's African American residents feel they're being left behind. US News and World Report, January 22, 2020

Wilson WJ: Another look at the truly disadvantaged. Polit Sci Q 106:639–656, 1991

Xue Y, Leventhal T, Brooks-Gunn J, Earls FJ: Neighborhood residence and mental health problems of 5- to 11-year-olds. Arch Gen Psychiatry 62:554–563, 2005

CHAPTER 8

Social Injustice and the Carceral System

LeRoy E. Reese, Ph.D.
Seyi O. Amosu, Ph.D.
Sarah Y. Vinson, M.D.

The "Criminal Justice" System

The criminal justice system is not *just*. It is, in fact, demonstrably unjust as to whom it criminalizes. This reality has led to a shift in its being referred to as the *carceral system*, which is the nomenclature used throughout this text. This issue of criminalization is often overlooked, with a focus on *who* is committing crime—and precluding critical examination of *how* crime is conceptualized and *what* the environmental contributors are. If the goal is a safer society, proactive, preventive approaches informed by the *how* and *what* can be taken to effectively reduce crime. In the United States, however, our systems default to reactive, punitive approaches (Robinson and Williams 2009). In order for a system to be just, legal consequences must be applied to all equitably (Robinson and Williams 2009). Ample evidence demonstrates that they are not. This injustice takes on heightened significance in the United States, given that the incarceration rate is the highest in the industrialized world (Meiners 2011).

The sheer volume of people with mental illnesses entangled in the carceral system makes knowledge of this system relevant to mental health professionals. Furthermore, it is a system that negatively impacts the mental health of individuals, families, and communities. In this chapter, we describe how the application of policies and laws and, in fact, the very construction of them disproportionately impact marginalized groups: Black people, those living in poverty, and people with serious mental illnesses.

Mass Incarceration and Inequity

The U.S. prison population has increased by 500% from approximately 100–200 per 100,000 adults in the 1970s to 700 per 100,000 adults in the present (Bark 2014; Wildeman and Wang 2017). This phenomenon, commonly referred to as *mass incarceration* (Tucker 2017), was not a function of increased criminal activity or improved crime-solving techniques over the past four decades. In fact, the number of people incarcerated for violent offenses has steadily declined during this time. Mass incarceration was, instead, a function of highly punitive, reactive policies that not only increased the reach of the carceral system but also racialized its impact (Alexander 2010).

It is no coincidence that rising incarceration coincided with a cluster of policies colloquially known as the "War on Drugs" (for an in-depth discussion, see Chapter 10, "Social Injustice and Substance Use Disorders"). These policy approaches were characterized by a significant shift in how drug-related offenses were classified, adjudicated, and sanctioned (Dumont et al. 2012). The Rockefeller Drug Laws, which were implemented in New York beginning in 1973, included long, harsh mandatory minimum sentences. For example, the mandatory minimum penalty for selling 2 ounces of an illicit substance (e.g., cocaine, marijuana, morphine) was increased to 15 years to life in prison—the same sentence imposed on a person found guilty of second-degree murder (Smith and Hattery 2010). The Rockefeller Drug Laws contained three policy approaches that were widely influential in shaping policies throughout the United States: 1) sentencing guidelines that took drug possession from a misdemeanor to a felony, 2) the possibility of life sentences for second or third felony convictions (or, as is more often the case, guilty pleas), and 3) differential sentencing for the sale or possession of crack cocaine versus powder cocaine (Smith and Hattery 2010).

Even though the two substances are nearly identical in chemical structure (Hart et al. 2014), possession of 5 grams of crack cocaine triggered the same minimum sentence as 500 grams of powder cocaine (Smith and Hattery

2010). The key differentiator was that the latter was associated with white people and the former with Black people. The policy's resultant racial inequity was stark: although Blacks and whites used cocaine at comparable rates, Blacks constituted more than 80% of those sentenced for cocaine-related offenses (Palamar et al. 2015). In practice, these policies criminalized substance use, and as a result, for many Black people, they also criminalized substance use disorders. More broadly, although white and Black people had similar rates of illicit drug use, Black people constituted 62% of individuals incarcerated in the War on Drugs (Dumont et al. 2012). Differential sentencing for certain drugs is one of many contributors to carceral system inequities. Another is differential perceptions of the dangerousness of different kinds of crime.

Public discourse and safety concerns are often focused on "street" crimes (e.g., burglary, theft, assault). This contrasts with the treatment of so-called white-collar crimes, which are sometimes portrayed as less serious even though "acts by the rich and powerful and by corporations produce far more damage to human life and property than all street crimes combined" (Robinson and Williams 2009, p. 11). Additionally, the socioeconomic status (middle and upper income) and race (white) of most who write and apply the laws are markedly different from the socioeconomic status (impoverished) and race and ethnicity (Black and brown, i.e., Latinx and Indigenous populations) of those who are most disproportionately judged by it (Robinson and Williams 2009). These group differences between the decision makers and defendants extend beyond race and income because people with mental illnesses as well as those who are undereducated or uneducated, gender nonconforming, and noncitizens are also vastly overrepresented in prison populations (Meiners 2011).

Notably, the demographics of groups that are overrepresented in the carceral system mirror those of groups underserved by the mental health care system. Specifically, low-income communities comprising largely ethnic minorities have less access to care for mental illnesses and substance use disorders (Dumont et al. 2012). In these same communities, overpolicing results in more ethnic minority people with untreated mental illnesses (and the concomitant impairment in judgment that may accompany it) having more interactions with law enforcement officers. In contrast, white people are more likely to receive treatment for substance use disorders (Dumont et al. 2012). Not surprisingly, inadequacies in mental health access persist behind bars. The high numbers of individuals with mental health and substance use disorders in need of treatment simply cannot be met in most correctional facilities (Hunt et al. 2015). Approximately half of all incarcerated persons have a mental illness of some kind, with 15%–20% having serious mental illnesses (Bark 2014).

Upstream Contributors to Inequity

The Juvenile Justice System

The two foremost stated purposes of the juvenile justice system are to 1) rehabilitate wayward youth through accountability and corrective training and 2) protect the larger society by providing a buffer between society and troubled youth who pose a danger to it (Alexander 2010; Zajac et al. 2015). In reality, the system often fails on both counts. Rather than promoting rehabilitation, institutional policies may result in retraumatization of an already highly traumatized group; up to 90% of justice-involved youth report prior trauma (Dierkhising et al. 2013). Furthermore, the system often is neither configured nor funded appropriately to meet the youth's mental health and substance use disorder treatment needs (Young et al. 2017). Additionally, juvenile justice becomes yet another source of structural trauma for children who have already been failed by one or more other highly influential systems: schooling, safety net, urban development, child welfare, or mental health care.

In some communities, educational systems may promote and perpetuate juvenile justice system involvement, feeding the school-to-prison pipeline (Kim et al. 2010; Mallett 2016). This process is characterized by punitive disciplinary policies that are inequitably applied to Black, brown, and poor students (Raufu 2017). These policies result in significant disparities in missed school days due to suspensions and expulsions for these students as compared with their nonmarginalized peers. This sets up students to fall behind academically (or further behind, as is often the case) and for being poorly supervised. It follows that there is a positive, direct correlation between missed school days and delinquent behaviors (Novak 2019). Additionally, substantial empirical literature describes increased mental illnesses and substance use disorders in justice-involved youth compared with youth who have no justice involvement (Voisin et al. 2017).

Given the reality of the reasons why youth are often detained, the system likely fares no better in achieving the second stated purpose of keeping society safe. The majority of justice-involved youth do not exhibit behaviors that pose a legitimate threat to society's safety. For many, their offenses are the result of poor supervision, a dearth of prosocial activities, and poverty—which could be considered the social determinants of delinquency (Spinney et al. 2016). The vast majority of youth in the juvenile justice system can be divided into three categories: those with truly criminogenic behaviors; those with a mental illness and associated problem behaviors; and those with mental illnesses, comorbid substance use disorders, and associated problem behaviors. In reality, it is these latter two groups that constitute the majority of system-involved youth (Spinney et al. 2016). The juvenile justice system frequently misses the valuable opportunity to rechart the course for youth by promoting their positive socioemotional development and addressing their mental health needs.

Instead, the juvenile justice system's current design allows the societal inequities that put youth at risk for involvement in the first place (e.g., limited family income, inadequate community resources, poor education and vocational opportunities) to further influence their trajectory in the juvenile and adult correctional systems (Anoshiravani 2020). For contrast, consider the case of a middle-class white teenager from a "good" neighborhood who uses marijuana. Given that he does not live in an overpoliced community, he may never be asked to empty his pockets, allowing his marijuana use to remain unknown to law enforcement. If drugs are somehow discovered on him, his local resources and his family's ability to hire a private attorney would provide him with concrete advantages throughout the adjudication process. These advantages might include relative ease in the creation of a plan, as an alternative to incarceration, that includes mental health treatment, access to private forensic mental health evaluators who could place the teenager's behavior in context, more hours and prioritization of his case by legal counsel, and family involvement unhindered by unreliable public transportation or lack of paid time off. He may also have a less problematic school disciplinary record because he had been appropriately tested and provided accommodations for his learning disorder in school. Racial bias may also play a role, as demonstrated by the fact that Black and brown youth are grossly overrepresented in the juvenile justice system even though they engage in similar kinds of criminal acts at rates comparable to that of their white peers (Morrow et al. 2015).

Functionally, the juvenile justice system serves as the middleman in the school-to-adult prison pipeline (Novak 2019). This reality promotes a developmental understanding of the highly cited statistic that one in three Black males are involved in the carceral system by age 35 (Taylor et al. 2018). It is a disservice to both the rehabilitation of youth and the safety of society (which also includes these youth and their families) to silo conversations about juvenile justice, inequities in the educational system, and social determinants of mental health driven by injustice. These structural issues are part of a self-perpetuating cycle. In communities disproportionately impacted by mass incarceration, the social fabric is frayed. Both the availability and the viability of young men as partners, husbands, parents, employees, and citizens are limited, creating debilitating burdens for many of the women and children in these communities. The next generation of youth, then, is disproportionately exposed to the social determinants of delinquency, including inadequate supervision and poverty.

Profit and Politics

Transinstitutionalization is a term often applied to the shunting of those individuals with serious mental illnesses from the mental health system into the carceral system. Policies started by Ronald Reagan's administration in the early 1980s and later amplified by Bill Clinton's administration fed the system another marginalized group—Black Americans. As stated by Michelle Alexander (2010), "The nature of the criminal justice system has changed. It is no longer primarily concerned with the prevention and punishment of crime, but rather with the management and control of the dispossessed" (p. 111). The subjugation of Black people by slavery and Jim Crow laws was transferred into the carceral system, largely facilitated by the War on Drugs. Predictably, with 500% more Americans incarcerated in the past several decades, more money is being spent by the government on incarceration, and businesses connected to the carceral system have made billions of dollars (Kaeble and Cowhig 2018; Sawyer and Wagner 2020). However, the design and maintenance of the carceral system are not simply a matter of politics and profit; they are also representative of systematic disenfranchisement—in effect, a structurally mediated assault against affected populations' economic and political power (Alexander 2010).

Rather than exacting justice and preserving community safety, the carceral system's policies and laws—and its selective implementation of them—perpetuate injustice and further destabilize vulnerable communities. Its immunity in doing so can be attributed, in no small part, to a highly effective cover story: one of protection from dangerous "others" such as criminalized Black people and "crazy, homicidal, maniac" people with mental illnesses. One need look no further than the misnomer commonly applied to this system: *criminal justice*. The dangerous other (criminal) leads it off, and a laudable outcome (justice) completes it. The messaging is powerful. Othering allows individuals in the broader society to believe that they are safely distanced from the system's reach, and the invocation of justice feeds presumptions that punishment is equitable. "Tough on crime" politicians ride this narrative into elected office with the vote of citizens who desire safety and with the campaign contributions of special interest groups such as bail bondsmen and private prison lobbyists. As an example, in the 2018 election cycle, one of these companies donated $1.2 million in the state of Florida alone (March 2018). These politicians' punitive policies continue the cycle of marginalization and selective criminalization. The disproportionately high rate of incarceration of Black people and people with mental illnesses creates and maintains public perception that these populations are dangerous and overly involved with criminal activities.

This phenomenon serves to amplify fear of these groups while diminishing empathy for them. Although public safety is undeniably a necessary and worthwhile pursuit, there are clear indicators that mass incarceration and the disproportionate incarceration of Black people and people with serious mental illnesses do not achieve that end. Most people with carceral system involvement have misdemeanor (or minor) charges (Sawyer and Wagner 2020). On any given day, more than 550,000 American citizens are held in jail because they cannot afford bail, not because they have been convicted of anything (Sawyer and Wagner 2020). For those who plead or are found guilty, longer sentences are actually associated with higher rates of recidivism (Mueller-Smith 2015). Furthermore, deprivation of liberty is not reserved for violent offenders; nearly half of state prison inmates and 92% of federal prison inmates are incarcerated for nonviolent offenses (Bronson and Carson 2017). Carceral system involvement does not reliably provide trajectory-transforming rehabilitative experiences, as demonstrated by the fact that 76% of released prisoners are rearrested within 5 years (Durose et al. 2014). Additionally, the mark of a felony conviction erects barriers in accessing gainful employment, which is a key factor in altering criminal behavior (Wadsworth 2001).

U.S. Department of Justice–funded research on previously incarcerated individuals demonstrated that quality job opportunities and labor force participation had direct and indirect effects on rates of both property and violent crimes (Wadsworth 2001). This effect was explained not only by unemployed individuals committing more crimes but by job market characteristics as well. Recidivism rates were lower for those individuals in school or with higher-quality jobs (Wadsworth 2001). These findings have clear implications for people with serious mental illnesses and Black people who are already disadvantaged in the job market because of stigma and racism (Bertrand and Mullainathan 2004; Stuart 2006). Being designated a convicted felon and/or having been convicted of a drug offense, even a misdemeanor, limits eligibility for federal educational financial aid (Federal Student Aid 2020), blocking paths to obtaining marketable skill sets. Individuals with the resilience and resourcefulness to overcome this initial barrier face yet another: the use of felony conviction inquiries to screen people out for many high-quality jobs—or any job, for that matter. Employment opportunities for formerly incarcerated people are dismally low (Western and Pettit 2002). Even after controlling for other relevant worker variables, research suggests that a history of incarceration can reduce an individual's wages later in life by 10%–30% (Western and Pettit 2002). The economic impact of incarceration serves to bolster the strong link between incarceration and economic disadvantage (Western and Pettit 2002).

In a country where health insurance coverage is frequently obtained as an employee benefit, unemployment and underemployment have significant implications for access to mental health care. Therefore, individuals who have been imprisoned—as discussed, a group that includes many Black people and people with serious mental illnesses—are at the mercy of government payers for insurance. Study results indicate that the number of persons diagnosed with serious mental illnesses in correctional facilities is more than three times the number in psychiatric hospitals (Torrey et al. 2010). The War on Drugs kicked off a trend of investments in incarceration and divestments in prevention and treatment. Antidrug allocations by the Department of Defense (DoD) and the Federal Bureau of Investigation (FBI) between 1981 and 1991 are illustrative: The DoD's antidrug allocations increased from $33 million to $1.042 billion, and the FBI's grew from $38 million to $181 million (Alexander 2010). In a legitimate war on drugs, it would follow that budgets for research, treatment, and prevention would also grow, or at the very least remain stable. However, during this same period in the 1980s, the federal government slashed funding to the National Institute on Drug Abuse (NIDA) and to antidrug programs in the Department of Education (Alexander 2010). This pattern of prioritizing punishment has persisted and is reflected in state spending as well. For example, during the economic downturn in 2009, funding within the control of state mental health authorities in the 50 states was reduced by $4.35 billion over 3 years (Lutterman 2012). A decline of this magnitude was not seen in state correctional spending. In fact, in 2010 nearly one out of three states *increased* their rates of correctional spending (Enns and Shanks-Booth 2015).

Disincentives for meaningful reform exist at multiple levels of government. Some counties take in substantial percentages of their total operating revenue from public safety and court fines. For example, 20% of the operating revenue in Ferguson, Missouri, was generated through public safety by disproportionately citing Black people (Maciag 2014). Also, states are allowed to take legal kickbacks from prison vendors that provide grossly overpriced services, such as charging up to $60 for a phone call (Raher 2020). Some have characterized this as a form of taxing inmates' families—a method of monetary redistribution from poor communities to wealthy corporations.

In addition, the Federal Bureau of Prisons boasts of its "positive [economic] impact on rural communities" (U.S. Department of Justice 2017). Notably, because prisons help rural communities' votes count more, those communities gain politically. Correctional facilities are located disproportionately in rural areas, whereas prisoners come disproportionately from urban areas (Porter et al. 2017). Even though prisoners cannot vote while imprisoned, counts of imprisoned people are used for congressional districting purposes. Furthermore, in 34 states, people with felony convictions cannot immediately vote after they have been released from prison. In effect, this results in a redistribution of political power to largely rural, conservative populations on the basis of a body count of a disenfranchised population (Alexander 2010).

Bending the Arc of the Carceral System Toward Justice

In its current state, the carceral system fails to stem the flow from the school-to-prison pipeline and saddles vulnerable populations with continued marginalization, disenfranchisement, and economic hardship. Frankly, it is hard to imagine a less therapeutic, more traumatizing system being permitted to shape so many lives and with such absolute authority—even to the point of condemnation to death. However, the carceral system is the closest thing to a functional safety net that exists in our society. It becomes a catch-all for people who fall through the cracks due to systemic failures in schooling, foster care, vocational opportunities, housing, and care for mental health and substance use disorders. Rather than being reliably provided with the resources needed for rehabilitation, individuals are subjected to a process that often yields poorer outcomes; amplifies preexisting stigmatization; fractures critical community connections; and is, by its punitive and arbitrary nature, traumatizing. For mental health professionals, especially those in public and community mental health, structural humility regarding the carceral system is a core competency. Once patients become probationers, parolees, or inmates, they are subjected to a litany of structural traumas. The carceral system threatens patients' security, autonomy, freedom, and relationships—all core elements of mental health and well-being.

Our society's problematic treatment of those ensnared by the carceral system is entrenched and multifaceted. Although certainly daunting, the breadth and variety of problems present myriad opportunities for improved practices, interventions, and policies. Every mental health professional has a role to play, whether it be as clinician, administrator, collaborator, or advocate (Vinson et al. 2020). Whereas mental illness carries a well-known stigma, incarceration comes not only with another mark against those affected but also with physical removal from natural supports and society, as well as, in many cases, legal removal from the voting booth. As clinicians, we should be informed about the system's inequities and injustices, be aware of the carceral system's reach in communities we serve, be curious about our patients' carceral system–associated traumas, and be internally reflective of our own biases against the criminalized other. As administrators, we can examine hiring and patient care policies for language that could differentially impact those with carceral system involvement, incorporate vocational training and support work as part of treatment, and partner with forensic peers who have lived experience with mental illnesses and have successfully reintegrated into society. As collaborators, we can work across disciplines through programs such as crisis intervention training and mental health courts. As advocates, we can push for reforms both as citizens and through mental health and medical professional organizations. Effective mental health promotion and patient-centered care not only require our awareness and acknowledgment of this system's impact on our patients' lives but also demand action within and across systems to mitigate these impacts.

Conclusion

Rectifying carceral system inequities will require a fundamental shift in society's perspective and approach. For many people, the carceral system provides a sense of security because the presence of prisons suggests the absence of criminals. However, this sense of security is false. A society without crime cannot be achieved by focusing on criminalized individuals. Instead, a truly safe society would need to intentionally address the structural framework for the conditions that create crime, such as institutional racism, poverty, poor educational and vocational opportunities, and untreated serious mental illnesses and substance use disorders. Meaningful change will occur only when social justice takes preeminence over criminal justice.

Questions for Self-Reflection

1. Which groups of people do I automatically associate with criminal behavior?
2. What associations do I have with people who participate in criminal behavior or illegal activity? What illegal activities have I participated in?
3. How do housing, education, and labor policies in my local community interface with the carceral system?

References

Alexander M: The New Jim Crow: Mass Incarceration in the Age of Colorblindness. New York, New Press, 2010

Anoshiravani A: Addressing the unmet health needs of justice system-involved youth. Lancet Public Health 5:e83, 2020

Bark N: Prisoner mental health in the USA. Int Psychiatry 11:53–55, 2014

Bertrand M, Mullainathan S: Are Emily and Greg more employable than Lakisha and Jamal? A field experiment on labor market discrimination. Am Econ Rev 94(4):991–1013, 2004

Bronson J, Carson EA: Prisoners in 2017. Washington DC, Bureau of Justice Statistics, 2017

Dierkhising CB, Ko SJ, Woods-Jaeger B, et al: Trauma histories among justice-involved youth: findings from the National Child Traumatic Stress Network. Eur J Psychotraumatol 4:20274, 2013

Dumont DM, Brockmann B, Dickman S, et al: Public health and the epidemic of incarceration. Annu Rev Public Health 33:325–339, 2012

Durose MR, Cooper AD, Snyder HN: Recidivism of Prisoners Released in 30 States in 2005: Patterns from 2005 to 2010. Washington, DC, Bureau of Justice Statistics, April 2014. Available at: www.bjs.gov/content/pub/pdf/rprts05p0510.pdf. Accessed April 20, 2020.

Enns P, Shanks-Booth D: The Great Recession and State Criminal Justice Policy: Do Economic Hard Times Matter? New York, Russell Sage Foundation, December 2015. Available at: www.russellsage.org/sites/all/files/Recession_Enns_Criminal.pdf. Accessed April 20, 2020.

Federal Student Aid: Eligibility for Students with Criminal Convictions. StudentAid.gov, 2020. Available at: https://studentaid.gov/understand-aid/eligibility/requirements/criminal-convictions. Accessed April 20, 2020.

Hart CL, Csete J, Habibi D: Methamphetamine: Fact vs. Fiction and Lessons from the Crack Hysteria. Washington, DC, Open Society Foundations, 2014. Available at: www.opensocietyfoundations.org/publications/methamphetamine-dangers-exaggerated. Accessed July 3, 2020.

Hunt E, Peters RH, Kremling J: Behavioral health treatment history among persons in the justice system: findings from the Arrestee Drug Abuse Monitoring II Program. Psychiatr Rehabil J 38:7–15, 2015

Kaeble D, Cowhig M: Correctional Populations in the United States, 2016. Washington, DC, Bureau of Justice Statistics, U.S. Department of Justice, Office of Justice Programs, 2018

Kim C, Losen DJ, Hewitt D: The School to Prison Pipeline: Structuring Legal Reform, New York, New York University Press, 2010

Lutterman T: The Impact of the State Fiscal Crisis on State Mental Health Systems. Winter 2011–2012 Update. Preliminary Results based on 41 States reporting. Alexandria, VA, NASMHPD Research Institute, March 2012. Available at: www.nri-inc.org/media/1102/2012-the-impact-of-the-state-fiscal-crisis-on-state-mental-health-systems-lutterman.pdf. Accessed Apr 26, 2020.

Maciag M: Skyrocketing court fines are major revenue generator for Ferguson. Folsom, CA, eRepublic, August 22, 2014. Available at: www.governing.com/topics/public-justice-safety/gov-ferguson-missouri-court-fines-budget.html. Accessed July 3, 2020.

Mallett CA: The school-to-prison pipeline: disproportionate impact on vulnerable children and adolescents. Educ Urban Soc 49:563–592, 2016

March W: Prison company bets big on Ashley Moody in Florida Attorney General race. Tampa Bay Times, October 26, 2018

Meiners ER: Ending the school-to-prison pipeline/building abolition futures. Urban Rev 43:547–565, 2011

Morrow WJ, Dario LM, Rodriguez N: Examining the prevalence of a 'youth discount' in the juvenile justice system. J Crime Justice 42:430–443, 2015

Mueller-Smith M: The Criminal Labor Market Impacts of Incarceration. Ann Arbor, Department of Economics, University of Michigan, August 18, 2015. Available at: https://sites.lsa.umich.edu/mgms/wp-content/uploads/sites/283/2015/09/incar.pdf. Accessed April 26, 2020.

Novak A: The school-to-prison pipeline: an examination of the association between suspension and justice system involvement. Crim Justice Behav 46:1165–1180, 2019

Palamar JJ, Davies S, Ompad DC, et al: Powder cocaine and crack use in the United States: an examination of risk for arrest and socioeconomic disparities in use. Drug Alcohol Depend 149:108–116, 2015

Porter SR, Voorheis JL, Sabol W: Correctional Facility and Inmate Locations: Urban and Rural Status Patterns. CARRA Working Paper Series Working Paper 2017-08. Washington, DC, Center for Administrative Records Research and Applications, U.S. Census Bureau, 2017

Raher S: The company store and the literally captive market: consumer law in prisons and jails. Hastings Race and Poverty Law Journal 17:1, 2020

Raufu A: School-to-prison pipeline: impact of school discipline on African American students. Journal of Education and Social Policy 1:47–53, 2017

Robinson M, Williams M: The myth of a fair criminal justice system. Justice Policy Journal 6:1–52, 2009

Sawyer W, Wagner P: Mass incarceration: the whole pie 2020. Northampton, MA, Prison Policy Initiative, March 24, 2020. Available at: www.prisonpolicy.org/reports/pie2020.html. Accessed April 20, 2020.

Smith E, Hattery AJ: African American men and the prison industrial complex. West J Black Stud 34:387, 2010

Spinney E, Yeide M, Feyerherm W, et al: Racial disparities in referrals to mental health and substance abuse services from the juvenile justice system: a review of the literature. J Crime Justice 39:153–173, 2016

Stuart H: Mental illness and employment discrimination. Curr Opin Psychiatry 19:522–526, 2006

Taylor RJ, Miller R, Mouzon D, et al: Everyday discrimination among African American men: the impact of criminal justice contact. Race Justice 8:154–177, 2018

Torrey EF, Kennard AD, Eslinger D, et al: More Mentally Ill Persons Are in Jails and Prisons than Hospitals: A Survey of the States. Alexandria, VA, Treatment Advocacy Center, May 2010. Available at: http://tulare.networkofcare.org/library/final_jails_v_hospitals_study1.pdf. Accessed April 26, 2018.

Tucker RB: The color of mass incarceration. Ethn Stud Rev 37–38:135–149, 2017

U.S. Department of Justice: FY 2016 Performance Budget Congressional Submission: Federal Prison System Buildings and Facilities. Washington, DC, U.S. Department of Justice, 2017

Vinson SY, Coffey TT, Jackson N, et al: Two systems, one population: achieving equity in mental healthcare for criminal justice and marginalized populations. Psychiatr Clin North Am 43(3)525–538, 2020

Voisin DR, Kim D, Takahashi L, et al: Involvement in the juvenile justice system for African American adolescents: examining associations with behavioral health problems. J Soc Serv Res 43:129–140, 2017

Wadsworth TP: Employment, crime, and context: a multi-level analysis of the relationship between work and crime. Doctoral dissertation, Seattle, University of Washington, 2001. Available at: www.ncjrs.gov/pdffiles1/nij/grants/198118.pdf. Accessed April 26, 2020.

Western B, Pettit B: Beyond crime and punishment: prisons and inequality. Contexts 1:37–43, 2002

Wildeman C, Wang EA: Mass incarceration, public health, and widening inequality in the USA. Lancet 389:1464–1474, 2017

Young S, Greer B, Church R: Juvenile delinquency, welfare, justice and therapeutic interventions: a global perspective. BJPsych Bull 41:21–29, 2017

Zajac K, Sheidow AJ, Davis M: Juvenile justice, mental health, and the transition to adulthood: a review of service system involvement and unmet needs in the U.S. Child Youth Serv Rev 56:139–148, 2015

CHAPTER 9

Social Injustice and the Health Care System

Michelle Ko, M.D., Ph.D.
Angie Lisbeth Cruz, M.H.S.
Janet R. Cummings, Ph.D.

The U.S. health care system both arose from and perpetuates long-standing structural conflicts (Stevens 2006). Medicine (and, more broadly, health care) is not separate from our society. Rather, as explained by historian Charles Rosenberg (2006), health care is "a fundamental social function [that] reflects, incorporates, and acts out more general aspects of social hierarchy, status, and power" (p. 23). In this chapter, we provide a brief overview of how structural inequities are re-created within three domains of the health care system: hospitals, physicians, and health insurance. We then explore two examples in depth—the affordability and geographic availability of mental health services—to illustrate these themes within mental health care.

Social Justice and the Health Care System

In the United States, the term health care system is widely understood to be a misnomer. The name implies the provision or maintenance of health, but providers and policies focus on the provision of clinical services. Likewise, care suggests that these services involve meeting the needs of patients, but services are more often centered on the arrangements of providers. Last, system implies an organized, cohesive, and connected structure, rather than the public-private patchwork of health system conglomerates, hospitals, clinics, private offices, and payers that is characteristic of health care in the United States today. Furthermore, to the extent that mental health services have been historically constructed as separate from medical services, the mental health care system is even more fragmented in addressing the mental health needs of the population. Thus, for the purposes of this discussion, we define *health care system* as the amalgamation of providers of clinical and social goods and services and the attendant payment and policies that support the continued operation of these providers. We provide a historical overview through a social justice lens of three major actors in this system: hospitals, the medical profession, and health insurance.

Hospitals

The history of health care in the United States is one of inequities that continue in the present. In her seminal work on the history of U.S. hospitals, Rosemary Stevens (1999) explained that the first inpatient care institutions were established as places of sick care for the poor, where individuals could live out a potentially terminal illness if they had no home or family to provide care. With the transformation of medicine to a scientific and technological enterprise, hospitals became institutions of treatment—a desirable place for care. Stevens described the rise of charitable hospitals, which served several social functions, including providing the upper class with public means to display their beneficence, while fostering the growth of institutions that did not have an explicit mission to serve vulnerable populations.

As in nearly all other sectors of society, racial segregation was a matter of course in U.S. hospitals. Construction of separate wards or denial of service to patients of color was routine and openly sanctioned until the Civil Rights Act of 1964 and the introduction of Medicare in 1965, which required hospital desegregation as a condition for reimbursement (Burrows and Berney 2019). Teaching hospitals, by contrast, were notable for their deliberate inclusion of patients marginalized by race and income—because "indigent patients were valuable cogs in the teaching-hospital machine" (Stevens 1999, p. 62).

However, fundamental causes of health inequities are replicated over time, even as the means change (Link and Phelan 1995). Despite the efforts to end de jure (legally sanctioned) segregation in the 1960s, hospitals and health systems continued de facto segregation by race and income, in part due to residential segregation of communities (Sarrazin et al. 2009). Regardless of federal requirements, hospitals located in affluent, predominantly white communities are typically physically distant from low-income communities of color, and the patient population of hospitals reflects the homogeneity of the surrounding service area.

Furthermore, private hospitals, whether for profit or not for profit, employ deliberate service and marketing strategies to reduce their exposure to low-income patients. For example, for-profit hospitals regularly eliminate unprofitable services that are disproportionately used by vulnerable populations, such as psychiatric emergency care (Horwitz 2005). At the same time, hospitals invest in technologies and amenities to appeal to more affluent communities, such as advanced imaging modalities. As a result, care for low-income communities of color is disproportionately concentrated in a subset of safety net hospitals that operate at zero or negative margins, have fewer resources for new capital such as health information technology, and are particularly dependent on government support (Hall 2012). Studies of safety net hospitals and those serving predominantly Black and/or minoritized populations have found mixed evidence on the quality of care provided by these institutions (Mouch et al. 2014). A major confounding factor is that these hospitals are serving populations with greater severity and complexity of illness.

As described by Camilleri (2018), in the past three decades, hospitals in low-income communities of color have been more likely to close, thus increasing strains on the remaining safety net providers. The Patient Protection and Affordable Care Act of 2010 (ACA) had the potential to bring much-needed financial relief to safety net hospitals by expanding insurance coverage for low-income populations, particularly through the Medicaid program. However, because not all states elected to expand Medicaid coverage, large disparities between hospitals emerged post-ACA. Those in expansion states have experienced substantial reductions in uncompensated care, whereas those in nonexpansion states have not; as a result, hospitals in nonexpansion states are facing increasing risk of closure (Camilleri 2018). Since the passage of the ACA, low-income communities of color have disproportionately borne the brunt of rural hospital closures (Thomas et al. 2019). Inequities in access to hospital care arise from the confluence of residential segregation, hospital imperatives to generate revenue, and state policy making.

Physicians

While hospitals were undergoing their technocratic transformation at the turn of the twentieth century, a parallel trend was playing out among physicians. The 1910 publication of the Flexner Report formalized medicine's evolution into a profession, calling for admissions standards, an emphasis on research and teaching, and the development of academic medical centers with full-time faculty (Miller and Weiss 2012). Arguing the need for technical standards in medical education, the Flexner Report also deliberately led to the dismantling of schools and hospitals that served Black and female medical students, who were otherwise excluded from the predominant institutions of the time (Barkin et al. 2010; Miller and Weiss 2012). For example, the Flexner Report's prioritization of physical facilities for conducting research and teaching brought attention to the inadequacies of the buildings used by Black medical schools. Rather than improve conditions and advance the education of Black and female medical students, the Flexnerian movement led to the closure of all existing Black medical schools except the Medical Department of Howard University and Meharry Medical College, as well as all but one of the women's medical colleges, Women's Medical College of Pennsylvania (Barkin et al. 2010; Miller and Weiss 2012).

At the same time, the American Medical Association (AMA) conducted stricter scrutiny of premedical education requirements and licensing (Miller and Weiss 2012). The AMA and the Association of American Medical Colleges (AAMC) pushed to increase premedical requirements for college-level coursework at a time when educational opportunities were restricted primarily to white men. In fact, only 3% of Black students in the South attended high school in 1910 (Miller and Weiss 2012). Furthermore, states began to require graduation from AMA-approved institutions for physician licensure. Thus, the physician pipeline was effectively constricted both before and after medical education.

Traditional medical schools would not be compelled to consider integration of racial and ethnic minority students until the civil rights movement prompted the AAMC to advance desegregation among its members in 1968. Following affirmative action initiatives, enrollment of Black students rose steadily and peaked in 1995 (Association of American Medical Colleges 2016). Then, starting with California in 1996, eight states banned their public institutions from considering race and ethnicity in admissions decisions, and many universities followed voluntarily. The share of underrepresented minorities in higher education plummeted, and the steady progress to diversify medicine came to a halt (Garces and Mickey-Pabello 2015). In 1996, 9% of all U.S. medical students were Black, versus 7% in 2019 (Association of American Medical Colleges 2016, 2019).

Compounding the lack of racial and ethnic diversity, the medical profession continues to reflect the consequences of economic and social inequality of the U.S. society at large. In 2019, only 5% of medical students reported parental incomes in the bottom quintile of U.S. households, versus 51% in the top quintile (Youngclaus and Roskovensky 2018). The physician workforce is a product of long-standing structured advantages, in which intergenerational wealth enables residence in communities with high-quality public education, purchase of private education, or both (Lucey and Saguil 2019). Children of educated parents are raised with the cultural capital and social networks needed to navigate elite college admissions and the costs of attendance, facilitating success in undergraduate years and medical school admissions. The trends started by Flexner—the emphasis on health technology through a research enterprise—have raised the costs of medical education (Miller and Weiss 2012). Rising debt among medical school graduates has garnered the lion's share of attention, but closer scrutiny reveals growing inequality: from 2010 to 2016, mean debt rose, but the percentage of graduates with zero debt also rose, from 16% to 27% (Grischkan et al. 2017). To the extent that structural racism denies socioeconomic privileges to racial and ethnic minorities, low-income minorities encounter the highest barriers to entering the medical profession (Lucey and Saguil 2019).

As a result of these socioeconomic inequities, physicians do not reflect the racial, ethnic, and sociodemographic characteristics of the populations they are serving. With insufficient diversity, the medical profession lacks the needed supply of physicians who are committed to working with underserved populations. Across decades of research, the most consistent predictor of practice in underserved communities, whether by race and ethnicity, income, or geography, is having a personal origin from one of those communities (Goodfellow et al. 2016). Physicians without such backgrounds are less likely to express interest in practicing in needed areas, and because of residential segregation, they may select practice locations that are inaccessible to underserved populations and that have no incentive to meet these populations' needs. Black and Latinx communities have fewer physicians across many specialties, from primary care to general surgery to medical subspecialties (Marrast et al. 2014). As discussed later in this chapter (see "Social Injustice and the Mental Health Care System"), accessibility barriers are particularly profound for office-based psychiatrists, who are both less likely to practice in minority communities and far less likely to accept insurance at all, much less public coverage (Bishop et al. 2014; Cummings 2015).

Furthermore, extensive examination of clinical encounters has found that racial, ethnic, linguistic, and cultural patient-physician concordance leads to improved communication and patient engagement (Shen et al. 2018). Lack of physician diversity contributes to patient reports of discrimination and medical mistrust, which in turn lead to fear of accessing care and reluctance to follow treatment recommendations (LaVeist et al. 2009). In summary, inequities in education, selection, and training in medicine culminate in a workforce that produces inequities in access to and quality of care.

Health Insurance Coverage

With the technocratic transformation in health care in the first half of the twentieth century, patients were increasingly unable to afford the new, scientifically based care. Access to care, therefore, depended on another relatively new development: health insurance. Initially, health insurance remained the purview of the few who were wealthy and worried enough to pay for individual coverage. During and immediately after World War II, the expansion of industrial manufacturing, combined with federal restrictions on raising wages, prompted employers to offer health insurance benefits as a nontaxed alternative to pay increases. From 1940 to 1950, the number of U.S. residents with private health insurance coverage ballooned from 20 million to 142 million; however, employer-sponsored coverage was concentrated among middle-class workers with skilled labor and white-collar occupations (Moseley 2018). Underlying structural processes such as underinvestment in K–12 education, job-location mismatch (in which jobs are located in areas far from communities of color), and hiring discrimination produce inequities in overall employment and types of employment on several intersecting dimensions, including gender, race, ethnicity, immigration status, and disability. Therefore, a system built on a foundation of private employer-based coverage reproduces inequities in health insurance.

Throughout the twentieth and twenty-first centuries, U.S. policy makers have considered multiple options to increase access to care. President Harry Truman advanced a proposal for a national health insurance program in 1947. The AMA launched vigorous opposition and garnered the support of Southern Democrats and a new Republican Congress, and the aim of universal coverage faded in 1948 (Oberlander 2003). The introduction of Medicare and Medicaid in 1965 brought coverage to older adults and to a subset of low-income parents, children, and people with disabilities, but objections of Southern Democrats and the AMA again blocked further expansion. In the intervening 45 years before the ACA, similar attempts, including from Presidents Nixon and Clinton, were handily dismantled by the same stakeholders. Thus, most low-income adults (with the exception of pregnant women) remained ineligible for Medicaid.

Within this historical context of failed attempts to expand coverage, the ACA was developed to meet expectations of political expediency. ACA supporters calculated that a series of policies built from the existing health care system would more likely receive bipartisan support from Congress than proposals that would abolish existing reimbursement structures (e.g., replacing private and public insurance with a national single-payer plan) (Skocpol 2010). Therefore, the ACA called for expanding coverage under the patchwork of public and private systems but included little to address the underlying drivers of inequities in coverage, distribution, and services. Nevertheless, 14 states, including some that blocked coverage expansions from the 1940s to 1990s, filed suit against the ACA, arguing that mandated coverage was unconstitutional (Kaiser Family Foundation 2020).

In 2012, the U.S. Supreme Court ruled that individually mandated coverage was permissible as a tax, whereas Medicaid expansion was unduly coercive to states. Thus, at the start of Medicaid expansion in 2014, only 25 states elected to do so (Kaiser Family Foundation 2020). The majority of Southern states declined expansion and instead pursued increasing restrictions on Medicaid eligibility, such as work requirements and time limits on benefits. Political science researchers have shown that the intersection of racial resentment among whites, low public support for Medicaid among white people, and a relatively larger Black population have driven state decisions not to expand Medicaid (Grogan and Park 2017). Racial animus, rather than party affiliation or ideology, has been consistently associated with opposition to the entire ACA (Maxwell and Shields 2014). As a result of political geography, the United States experienced widening inequities in coverage. In 2019, the percentage of uninsured residents in nonexpansion states was nearly double that of expansion states (18.5% vs. 9.6%) (Garfield et al. 2020).

One of the consequences of the ongoing failure to ensure health care coverage for all U.S. residents is persistent racial and ethnic inequities in insurance coverage. Structural racism has produced barriers to jobs with health insurance benefits for Black and Latinx populations and relegated their opportunities to lower-wage jobs. As a result, Black and Latinx people are disproportionately represented among the uninsured and those with Medicaid coverage (Artiga et al. 2020).

Social Injustice and the Mental Health Care System

Structural inequities over time have produced racial and socioeconomic inequities within the health care system at large, and similar conditions are repeated and amplified for those with mental health conditions and substance use disorders. In 2018, among Black adults with any mental illness, 69% received no treatment, including 42% of those with severe mental illness; for Latinx adults, lack of treatment is comparable, at 67% and 44%, respectively (Substance Abuse and Mental Health Services Administration 2019). For those with substance use disorders, these gaps are even starker, with 88% and 89% of Black and Latinx adults, respectively, reporting no treatment.

We draw on dimensions from Penchansky and Thomas's (1981) framework on access to care to highlight how structural conditions have contributed to inequities in access to mental health services. See Table 9–1 for dimensions and definitions of health care access as described within that framework.

In the following subsections, we focus on the dimensions of affordability, accessibility, and availability of mental health care services. Barriers associated with these domains of access can interact and compound one another, manifesting as disparities in access by race, ethnicity, and income.

Mental Health Services and Affordability

Barriers related to affordability are exacerbated in the mental health care system relative to other sectors of health care. First, coverage for mental health services and substance use treatment has been historically less generous than coverage for other conditions, leading to greater numbers of uninsured and underinsured for mental health treatment. Second, in the absence of broad-based private coverage, Medicaid has assumed a critical role in mental health coverage, especially for individuals with serious mental illnesses. Federal and state decisions about who is eligible for Medicaid coverage are highly consequential for those with mental health and substance use disorders.

Insurance Coverage and Access to Mental Health Services

From the 1960s to 1970s, private and public coverage expanded for inpatient psychiatric care but not outpatient services (Mechanic and Grob 2006). Health insurance plans capped coverage for outpatient mental health services in numerous ways, such as by limiting the number of visits or days; offering lower reimbursement rates; imposing cost sharing; setting benefit limits; or, in the case of substance use disorder treatment, providing no coverage at all (Cummings et al. 2013a). Congress passed successive laws in 1996, 2008, and 2010 (as part of the ACA) to close the gaps in coverage, but exceptions remain (Cummings et al. 2013a). For example, requirements apply only to individual and small-group markets, not to large-group plans or to self-insured plans offered by large employers. Post-ACA trends suggest that coverage discrepancies could be narrowing, but only

TABLE 9–1. Penchansky and Thomas's framework on access to care

Dimension	Definition
Affordability	Prices and providers' payment requirements in relation to patients' income, ability to pay, and health insurance
Availability	Adequacy of supply of facilities and providers in a given geographic area
Accessibility	Relationship between the location of patients and the location of health care facilities and providers (accounting for travel distance, time, and cost)
Accommodation	Methods of organization of health care resources for patients (e.g., hours of operation) and alignment of resources with patients' needs and ability to access them
Acceptability	Patients' attitudes about provider characteristics and the providers' practices and perceptions of the patients they serve

Source. Penchansky and Thomas 1981.

because private insurers are requiring more cost sharing across the board (National Academies of Sciences, Engineering, and Medicine 2018).

In addition, reimbursement for mental health services is lower than that for other health care services. In 2015, other physicians received 14%–20% higher payments than psychiatrists for visits of comparable complexity (Melek et al. 2017). With lower reimbursement rates and restrictions on services, it is unsurprising that as of 2009–2010, nearly half of office-based psychiatrists opted out of private insurance networks entirely (Bishop et al. 2014). However, the data used in this study did not provide information about the extent to which some psychiatrists were employed in multiple jobs (e.g., operating a private practice and working in the public sector). The proportion of mental and behavioral health services received out of network was 3.6–5.8 times higher than other medical and surgical services (Melek et al. 2017). When providers decline to accept insurance payments, the financial resources needed to access care increase several times over.

With constraints on both coverage and the supply of providers who will accept that coverage, access to mental health services has been narrowed to individuals with the financial means to pay a substantial part of, or all, out-of-pocket costs for care. In 2011, of the non–older adult respondents to the National Survey on Drug Use and Health who had any mental illness, only 25% of the uninsured received any treatment; of those with private insurance, treatment increased only modestly to 38% (Walker et al. 2015). Because structural inequities have fostered a system in which people of color have lower average incomes, affordability issues contribute to racial inequities in access to mental health services. Among Black adults who reported unmet needs for mental health treatment, cost was reported twice as often as minimization of symptoms and nearly five times as often as stigma as the most common reason for not seeking care (Alang 2019).

Medicaid and Mental Health Services

In the absence of broad coverage, Medicaid has become an especially important payer of mental health services, especially for individuals with the most severe mental health disorders (Buck et al. 2000). Individuals with mental health and substance use conditions have higher rates of poverty and disability and thus are more likely to be eligible for Medicaid. In 2016, Medicaid covered 9.1 million adults with mental illnesses—21% of all noninstitutionalized adults with any mental illness and 26% of those with serious mental illness (Zur 2017). Medicaid accounted for 25% of U.S. spending on mental health services in 2014 (Mark et al. 2016). As stated earlier in this chapter (see "Health Insurance Coverage"), people of color are disproportionately represented within the Medicaid population.

Given the outsized role that Medicaid plays in affordability of mental health services, access depends on state policy decisions on eligibility. In states that elected to implement Medicaid expansion under the ACA, low-income adults with mental health needs, and particularly people of color, experienced substantial gains in coverage (Lipton et al. 2019). Multiple studies found that expanding Medicaid coverage increased access to mental health and substance use disorder treatment (Finkelstein et al. 2012; Wen et al. 2015). States that expanded Medicaid coverage witnessed increases in prescriptions and treatment for opioid use disorders (Antonisse et al. 2017). Conversely, the net implication of Medicaid expansion studies is that low-income adults in nonexpansion states remain uninsured and underinsured for mental health services. Given the racialized political dynamics with respect to states' decisions on Medicaid eligibility, the result is inequities in affordability by geography. The case of Medicaid, a core component of mental health and substance use treatment, also illustrates how structural racism produces barriers to care for whites as well as people of color.

Geographic Accessibility and Availability of Outpatient Mental Health Services

Penchansky and Thomas (1981) described two dimensions of health care access—accessibility and availability—that further capture how health care resources are distributed by geography at the local level (see Table 9–1).

Many of the same historical and social forces that produce inequities in the geographic distribution of health care system resources in general may apply to mental health care services.

Deinstitutionalization and the Emergence of Outpatient Specialty Mental Health Care

Accessibility and availability first must be understood through the historical context of how outpatient mental health care services emerged in the United States. The first steps began in the 1950s to 1960s with deinstitutionalization, the shifting of care of people with serious mental illnesses from residential institutions to community settings (Mechanic and Grob 2006). Proponents called for deinstitutionalization in part because of the efficacy of new psychotherapeutic medications, as well as growing concerns over patient safety in state mental hospitals. However, when they called for community-based care, they assumed that the community had mental health care providers, in addition to adequate housing and family and social support—an assumption unfounded in low-income communities (Mechanic and Grob 2006).

The Community Mental Health Act of 1963 provided subsidies for the construction of outpatient community mental health centers, but local communities bore the responsibility of raising funds for day-to-day operations. The act also offered no provisions to grow the psychiatry workforce needed to staff community mental health centers. The Carter administration attempted to address these gaps through the Mental Health Services Act of 1980, only to have the legislation be immediately repealed by the Reagan administration in 1981 (Mechanic and Grob 2006).

Currently, there are at least two separate outpatient specialty mental health systems. One system comprises solo and small group practices, including psychiatrists and therapists with master's and doctoral degrees. This group is more likely to be located in higher-income communities (Cummings et al. 2017). The presence of a wealthier patient base also makes it feasible to choose not to accept insurance because this population is most likely able to pay the full cost of care without the need for insurance support. Medicaid participation among psychiatrists is especially low and declining. As of 2015, only 35% of office-based psychiatrists accepted Medicaid (Wen et al. 2015).

The second system includes specialty outpatient mental health treatment facilities, which offer a structured service setting or program that provides ambulatory mental health care. These specialty outpatient facilities can be publicly or privately owned, and they play a critical role within the continuum of mental health care services for two key reasons (Cummings et al. 2013b). First, they typically offer a breadth of services for individuals with acute and persistent mental health needs, including psychotropic medication management, individual psychotherapy, family and group therapy, and supportive services such as case management and peer services (Substance Abuse and Mental Health Services Administration 2018). Second, in contrast to solo or small group practices, the vast majority of these facilities are financially accessible to people with public insurance (Jacobs et al. 2005) and part of the safety net system. Safety net providers deliver significant health care to vulnerable patients, including those who qualify for Medicaid or are uninsured (Institute of Medicine 2000). According to a 2017 survey, 94% of outpatient mental health treatment facilities accepted Medicaid (Substance Abuse and Mental Health Services Administration 2018).

Geographic Access to Outpatient Mental Health Services

Research has documented socioeconomic inequities in geographic access to mental health services in private solo or small group practices. These smaller practices of mental health specialists are more likely to be located in higher-income than in lower-income communities. In contrast, specialty outpatient mental health treatment facilities are more likely to be located in lower-income compared with higher-income communities (Cummings et al. 2017). Geographic access is especially important for low-income communities because many residents also encounter barriers related to transportation (Syed et al. 2013).

A growing body of evidence has documented persistent inequities in geographic access to mental health services both in private solo or small group practices and in the mental health safety net. Consistent with studies on providers in other specialties, a study by Cummings et al. (2017) found that psychiatrists and therapists were less likely to be located in communities with high percentages of Black and Latinx residents (>25% and 50%, respectively) than in communities with less than 1% of residents from either group. Earlier research has likewise shown that Black and Latinx communities, and particularly those with greater levels of residential segregation, have fewer available mental health providers (Dinwiddie et al. 2013).

Outpatient mental health treatment facilities are also less likely to be located in communities of color. Counties with a higher percentage of Black and Latinx residents are significantly less likely to have a facility that accepts Medicaid, even after controlling for poverty and rurality (Cummings et al. 2013a, 2017). Moreover, outpatient mental health treatment facilities are also less likely to be located in smaller communities (i.e., zip code tabulation areas) with >50% Black and Latinx residents than in communities with <1% of residents from either group, respectively (Cummings et al. 2017).

The literature to date has not explicitly tested the mechanisms to explain why these communities of color experience shortages of the very safety net providers intended to make up for private sector inequities. Limited federal investment in the outpatient mental health care safety net may be a contributing factor. In contrast to primary care community health centers, outpatient mental health facilities operate without additional federal grants or reimbursements and receive little attention or support for quality improvement. Because federal investment in the outpatient mental health care safety net is limited, mental health facilities may be unable or unwilling to operate in the same way that community health centers operate, thus being less likely to exist in communities of color.

Conclusion

Structural inequities shape the affordability, accessibility, and availability of mental health services in the United States. These barriers intersect with structural and institutional racism to produce even greater inequities for communities of color. In their review of deinstitutionalization, Mechanic and Grob (2006) described the consequences of moving services to persistently underresourced community settings: a rise in homelessness, substance use disorders, and admissions to nursing homes, along with the criminalization of people with mental illnesses. They coined the term transinstitutionalization because individuals with severe mental illnesses were simply shifted from one institutional setting to another. Unfortunately, none of these alternative institutional settings have been properly equipped to provide adequate services to the populations most in need of accessible, high-quality mental health care.

Questions for Self-Reflection

1. If I have mental health care coverage, how good is this coverage? How does my own health care coverage improve or exacerbate mental health inequities?
2. What decisions went into my choosing what type of mental health care delivery system to practice in?
3. What was my state's decision regarding Medicaid expansion? How has this decision impacted my patients, if at all?

References

Alang SM: Mental health care among blacks in America: confronting racism and constructing solutions. Health Serv Res 54:346–355, 2019

Antonisse L, Garfield R, Rudowitz R, Artiga S: The Effects of Medicaid Expansion Under the ACA: Updated Findings From a Literature Review. San Francisco, CA, Kaiser Family Foundation, 2017

Artiga S, Orgera K, Damico A: Changes in Health Coverage by Race and Ethnicity since the ACA, 2010–2018. San Francisco, CA, Kaiser Family Foundation, March 5, 2020. Available at: www.kff.org/disparities-policy/issue-brief/changes-in-health-coverage-by-race-and-ethnicity-since-the-aca-2010-2018/. Accessed May 1, 2020.

Association of American Medical Colleges: Longitudinal Applicant, Matriculant, Enrollment, and Graduation Tables. Washington, DC, AAMC Diversity, 2016. Available at: www.aamcdiversityfactsandfigures2016.org/report-section/applicants-enrollment/#tablepress-3a. Accessed May 1, 2020.

Association of American Medical Colleges: FACTS: Applicants, Matriculants, Enrollment, Graduates, MD–PhD, and Residency Applicants Data. Washington, DC, Association of American Medical College, 2019. Available at: www.aamc.org/data/facts. Accessed May 1, 2020.

Barkin SL, Fuentes-Afflick E, Brosco JP, Tuchman AM: Unintended consequences of the Flexner report: women in pediatrics. Pediatrics 126:1055–1057, 2010

Bishop TF, Press MJ, Keyhani S, Pincus HA: Acceptance of insurance by psychiatrists and the implications. JAMA Psychiatry 71:176–181, 2014

Buck J, Miller K, Bae J: Mental health and substance use services in Medicaid, 1986–1992. Rockville, MD, Substance Abuse and Mental Health Services Administration, 2000

Burrows V, Berney B: Creating equal health opportunity: how the medical civil rights movement and the Johnson administration desegregated U.S. hospitals. J Am Hist 105:885–911, 2019

Camilleri S: The ACA Medicaid expansion, disproportionate share hospitals, and uncompensated care. Health Serv Res 53:1562–1580, 2018

Cummings JR: Rates of psychiatrists' participation in health insurance networks. JAMA 313:190–191, 2015

Cummings JR, Lucas SM, Druss BG: Addressing public stigma and disparities among persons with mental illness: the role of federal policy. Am J Public Health 103:781–785, 2013a

Cummings JR, Wen H, Ko M, Druss BG: Geography and the Medicaid mental health care infrastructure: implications for health care reform. JAMA Psychiatry 70:1084–1090, 2013b

Cummings JR, Allen L, Clennon J, et al: Geographic access to specialty mental health care across high- and low-income U.S. communities. JAMA Psychiatry 74:476–484, 2017

Dinwiddie GY, Gaskin DJ, Chan KS, et al: Residential segregation, geographic proximity and type of services used: evidence for racial/ethnic disparities in mental health. Soc Sci Med 80:67–75, 2013

Finkelstein A, Taubman S, Wright B, et al: The Oregon Health Insurance Experiment: evidence from the first year. Q J Econ 127:1057–1106, 2012

Garces LM, Mickey-Pabello D: Racial diversity in the medical profession: the impact of affirmative action bans on underrepresented study of color matriculation in medical schools. J Higher Educ 86:264–294, 2015

Garfield R, Orgera K, Damico A: The Coverage Gap: Uninsured Poor Adults in States That Do Not Expand Medicaid. San Francisco, CA, Kaiser Family Foundation, January 14, 2020. Available at: www.kff.org/medicaid/issue-brief/the-coverage-gap-uninsured-poor-adults-in-states-that-do-not-expand-medicaid. Accessed May 1, 2020.

Goodfellow A, Ulloa JG, Dowling PT, et al: Predictors of primary care physician practice location in underserved urban or rural areas in the United States: a systematic literature review. Acad Med 91:1313–1321, 2016

Grischkan J, George BP, Chaiyachati K, et al: Distribution of medical education debt by specialty, 2010–2016. JAMA Intern Med 177:1532–1535, 2017

Grogan CM, Park SE: The racial divide in state Medicaid expansions. J Health Polit Policy Law 42:539–572, 2017

Hall MA: Health Care Safety Net Resources by State. Winston-Salem, NC, Robert Wood Johnson Foundation, 2012

Horwitz JR: Making profits and providing care: comparing nonprofit, for-profit, and government hospitals. Health Aff 24:790–801, 2005

Institute of Medicine: America's Health Care Safety Net: Intact but Endangered. Edited by Lewin ME, Altman S; Committee on the Changing Market, Managed Care, and the Future Viability of Safety Net Providers. Washington, DC, National Academies Press, 2000

Jacobs S, Wilk J, Chen D, et al: Datapoints: Medicaid as a payer for services provided by psychiatrists. Psychiatr Serv 56:1356, 2005

Kaiser Family Foundation: Status of State Action on the Medicaid Expansion Decision. San Francisco, CA, Kaiser Family Foundation, February 19, 2020. Available at: www.kff.org/health-reform/state-indicator/state-activity-around-expanding-medicaid-under-the-affordable-care-act/?currentTimefra. Accessed May 1, 2020

LaVeist TA, Isaac LA, Williams KP: Mistrust of health care organizations is associated with underutilization of health services. Health Serv Res 44:2093–2105, 2009

Link BG, Phelan J: Social conditions as fundamental causes of disease. J Health Soc Behav 20:80–94, 1995

Lipton BJ, Decker SL, Sommers BD: The Affordable Care Act appears to have narrowed racial and ethnic disparities in insurance coverage and access to care among young adults. Med Care Res Rev 76:32–55, 2019

Lucey CR, Saguil A: The consequences of structural racism on MCAT scores and medical school admissions: the past is prologue. Acad Med 95:351–356, 2019

Mark TL, Yee T, Levit KR, et al: Insurance financing increased for mental health conditions but not for substance use disorders, 1986–2014. Health Aff 35:958–965, 2016

Marrast LM, Zallman L, Woolhandler S, et al: Minority physicians' role in the care of underserved patients: diversifying the physician workforce may be key in addressing health disparities. JAMA Intern Med 174:289–291, 2014

Maxwell A, Shields T: The fate of Obamacare: racial resentment, ethnocentrism and attitudes about healthcare reform. Race Soc Probl 6:293–304, 2014

Mechanic D, Grob GN: Rhetoric, realities, and the plight of the mentally ill in America, in History and Health Policy in the United States: Putting the Past Back In. Edited by Stevens CE, Rosenberg LR, Burns LR. New Brunswick, NJ, Rutgers University Press, 2006, pp 229–255

Melek SP, Perlman D, Davenport S: Addiction and Mental Health vs. Physical Health: Analyzing Disparities in Network Use and Provider Reimbursement Rates. Milliman Research Report. Washington, DC, Milliman, 2017

Miller LE, Weiss RM: Revisiting black medical school extinctions in the Flexner era. J Hist Med Allied Sci 67:217–243, 2012

Moseley GB: The U.S. health care non-system, 1908–2008. Virtual Mentor 10:324–331, 2018

Mouch CA, Regenbogen SE, Revels SL, et al: The quality of surgical care in safety net hospitals: a systematic review. Surgery 155:826–838, 2014

National Academies of Sciences, Engineering, and Medicine: Health-Care Utilization as a Proxy in Disability Determination. Washington DC, National Academies Press, 2018

Oberlander J: The Political Life of Medicare. Chicago, IL, University of Chicago Press, 2003

Penchansky R, Thomas J: The concept of access: definition and relationship to consumer satisfaction. Med Care 19:127–140, 1981

Rosenberg CE: Anticipated consequences: historians, history and health policy, in History and Health Policy in the United States: Putting the Past Back In. Edited by Stevens CE, Rosenberg LR, Burns LR. New Brunswick, NJ, Rutgers University Press, 2006, pp 13–31

Sarrazin MS, Campbell ME, Richardson KK, Rosenthal GE: Racial segregation and disparities in health care delivery: conceptual model and empirical assessment. Health Serv Res 44:1424–1444, 2009

Shen MJ, Peterson EB, Costas-Muniz R, et al: The effects of race and racial concordance on patient-physician communication: a systematic review of the literature. J Racial Ethn Health Disparities 5:117–140, 2018

Skocpol T: The political challenges that may undermine health reform. Health Aff 29:1288–1292, 2010

Stevens RA: In Sickness and in Wealth: American Hospitals in the Twentieth Century. Baltimore, MD, Johns Hopkins University Press, 1999

Stevens RA: Introduction, in History and Health Policy in the United States: Putting the Past Back In. Edited by Stevens CE, Rosenberg LR, Burns LR. New Brunswick, Rutgers University Press, 2006, pp 1–12

Substance Abuse and Mental Health Services Administration: National Mental Health Services Survey (N-MHSS): 2017, Data on Mental Health Treatment Facilities. Rockville, MD, Substance Abuse and Mental Health Services Administration, 2018

Substance Abuse and Mental Health Services Administration: Key Substance Use and Mental Health Indicators in the United States: Results from the 2018 National Survey on Drug Use and Health. Rockville, MD, Substance Abuse and Mental Health Services Administration, 2019

Syed S, Gerber B, Sharp L: Traveling towards disease: transportation barriers to health care access. J Community Health 38:976–993, 2013

Thomas SR, Pink GH, Reiter KL: Characteristics of Communities Served by Rural Hospitals Predicted to Be at High Risk of Financial Distress in 2019. Chapel Hill, NC, Rural Health Research Program, 2019

Walker ER, Cummings JR, Hockenberry JM, Druss BG: Insurance status, use of mental health services, and unmet need for mental health care in the United States. Psychiatr Serv 66:578–584, 2015

Wen H, Druss BG, Wilk A, Cummings JR: Effect of Medicaid expansions on health insurance coverage and access to care among low-income adults with behavioral health conditions. Health Serv Res 50:1787–1809, 2015

Youngclaus J, Roskovensky L: An updated look at the economic diversity of U.S. medical students. AAMC Anal Brief 18:1–3, 2018

Zur J: Medicaid's Role in Financing Behavioral Health Services for Low-Income Individuals. San Francisco, CA, Kaiser Family Foundation, 2017

PART III
DIAGNOSES AND CONDITIONS

CHAPTER 10

Social Injustice and Substance Use Disorders

Jessica Isom, M.D., M.P.H.
Sonya M. Shadravan, M.D.
Melvin Wilson, M.B.A., L.C.S.W.

The treatment of people with substance use disorders, by both broader society and the health care system, epitomizes the interface of injustice and illness. This *mis*treatment has been more influenced by public narratives based on stigma, racism, and classism than by professional knowledge based on scientific literature or best practices. Conceptualizations of criminality, violence, morality, and free will have also factored prominently. Correspondingly, health and legal policies have been shaped primarily by societal messaging and economic and political incentives rather than biological, medical, or epidemiological data (Barnes and Kingsnorth 1996). Although the demographics and substances of drug epidemics in the United States have differed across time, the societal response is reliably shaped by key factors: stigma, media portrayals influenced by social hierarchies, inequities in treatment, and the racialization and criminalization of substance use. In this chapter, we explore these key factors, including their intersection with the "War on Drugs" and their collective influence on the opioid and cocaine epidemics.

Substance Use Disorders and Society

Stigma

Stigma can be conceptualized as an interplay between power and negative stereotyping, resulting in a devalued group of people who are vulnerable to marginalization (Link and Phelan 2001). This process includes the labeling of a distinguishable group, the association of this group with undesirable characteristics, a clear demarcation of *us* versus *them*, and the resulting status loss and discrimination experienced by the targeted group. Both in the general public and within health care settings, the level of stigma experienced by people with substance use disorders is substantial. In fact, stigma and discrimination against people with substance use disorders are even greater than against people with other psychiatric disorders—an already highly stigmatized group (Yang et al. 2017).

Stigma is a potent barrier to recognition and treatment of substance use disorders. *Public stigma*—stereotypes about moral weakness and dangerousness of people with substance use disorders—influences how people entrusted with their care *think* about them, and *enacted stigma*—manifestations of public stigma, including discrimination and marginalization—influences how people entrusted with their care *relate* to them (Tsai et al. 2019). Public stigma, often driven by media portrayals and anecdotes about people with substance use disorders, leads to enacted stigma, shaping clinical encounters, resource allocation, and care provision—or lack thereof. The combination of public stigma and enacted stigma results in *structural stigma*, in which discrimination is codified into laws, norms, and policies that ultimately harm people with substance use disorders (Tsai et al. 2019).

Structural stigma is a root cause of the segregation of substance use disorder services from other health care services. People with substance use disorders are depicted as morally and spiritually bankrupt and often as criminals. Ideally, the health care system would employ medical knowledge to counter these depictions; instead, it has abdicated responsibility for what is indisputably a health issue, outsourcing treatment options to churches and prisons (Office of the Surgeon General 2016).

Media Portrayals

Media serves as a conduit for public stigma. As a result, it holds great power. Popular portrayals of particular substances used by particular groups of people at particular times, often under the guise of authoritative medical science, have potent downstream impacts on health and legal policy. In turn, policy reverberates through communities, interfacing with social systems and impacting poverty, employment, immigration, housing, child welfare, and access to food (Drucker 2011). Importantly, these dynamic racialized narratives are very often divorced from the medical knowledge of their era or the true demographics of people who use substances.

There is a strong relationship between the tone and content of media coverage and the class and race of the population covered. Substances associated with citizens who are valued by society are reported on differently than substances associated with citizens who are stigmatized and oppressed (Netherland and Hansen 2016). In turn, public discourse, which is informed by this media coverage, influences the responses of health care leaders and lawmakers. In some instances, this response can be characterized as a drug-related moral panic, which develops when a deviance label is applied to a target population while structural factors are hidden. In addition to further stigmatizing the targeted group, this moral panic distracts policy makers from structural interventions that would more effectively address the problem (Eversman and Bird 2017). Moral panic holds significant implications for treatment. The media response to the 1980s cocaine epidemic in urban Black communities and to the current opioid epidemic in middle-class white communities is highly illustrative of this phenomenon.

Conversations about "crack mothers" and "crack babies" revolved around the moral depravity of addiction, nearly robbing both parent and child of their humanity (Logan 1999). The damning characterization of Black women choosing the crack pipe over motherhood was grossly oversimplified, failing to consider professional knowledge of etiologies and the course of substance use disorders. These portrayals are in stark contrast to the humanizing, contextualized media coverage of the genetic, environmental, structural, psychological, and policy-related contributions to the opioid epidemic. Discourse analyses of the news coverage narrating the current opioid epidemic are telling in that they reflect the privilege of whiteness, geography, and class as protective barriers against less empathic media coverage (Netherland and Hansen 2016). The result has been sympathetic policy makers advancing nonpunitive approaches to curtailing the tide of opioid misuse.

Inequities in Treatment

On the basis of the interplay of media depictions and policy, predictably, race and class factor prominently in care. Race is operationalized as a privilege or barrier, resulting in inequitable outcomes for people with substance use disorders. The primary source for these inequities is structural—not the result of individual or cultural behaviors. Treatment is extremely difficult to access, and even when treatment is available, it is often siloed. On the basis of medical knowledge, such an approach precludes optimal care. Substance use disorders have significant comorbidity with many chronic diseases, and there is ample evidence that integrated care approaches improve the management of chronic illnesses, substance use disorders included (Office of the Surgeon General 2016). The relationship between stigma and inequity in health care is demonstrated by the inadequate training of health professionals, misdiagnosis of patients, discriminatory institutional practices experienced by patients with substance use disorder diagnoses, and provision of suboptimal health care for people with substance use disorders (Office of the Surgeon General 2016; van Boekel et al. 2013).

Additionally, people in need of care are well aware of the consequences of marginalization that result from being labeled as an "addict." This is a key contributor to patients' documented aversion to disclosing their substance misuse to health care professionals (McNeely et al. 2018). Their reluctance to do so, while understandable, presents a barrier to identification and treatment. Provider misperceptions about the treatability of substance use disorders present yet another impediment. People with substance use disorders *do* suffer from a chronic relapsing course of illness; however, the notion that substance use disorders have a more complex course than other chronic illnesses is not based in evidence. In fact, the relapse rate for substance use disorders is comparable to that for hypertension, diabetes mellitus, and asthma (McLellan et al. 2000). Stigma held by providers disincentivizes the provision of care and can result in confirmation bias when relapses occur.

Furthermore, criminalization contributes to vast undertreatment and exacerbation of substance use disorders and other common comorbidities, such as PTSD (Roberts et al. 2015). In a 2013 study, more than 50% of incarcerated adults met DSM-IV (American Psychiatric Association 1994) criteria for drug abuse or dependence, as compared with 5%–13% in community populations (Belenko et al. 2013). Despite this high prevalence, only 6%–10% of incarcerated persons with substance use disorders reported receiving any clinical treatment while incarcerated, and less than 25% reported having *ever* received outpatient treatment in the community (Belenko et al. 2013). Although significant evidence exists for the efficacy of many treatment modalities, including medication-assisted treatment, these are rarely used in carceral settings (Belenko et al. 2013).

Social and treatment services often must compete for funding allocation during state and local budget processes. Therefore, when substance use treatment is incorporated into carceral settings, the funding of public resources, including community mental health treatment, can suffer

(Drucker 2011). Also, this approach does nothing to address the underlying problem of ensnaring individuals with a serious health need in the inherently punitive carceral system. Although diversion programs have the potential to address racially inequitable access to mental health services (Appel et al. 2020), they are often disproportionately offered to white defendants (Barnes and Kingsnorth 1996). As Drucker (2011) described in *A Plague of Prisons*, "the fundamental clinical accountability of drug treatment professionals to individual patients has been subordinated to the goals of the criminal justice system" (p. 57).

Criminalization and Racialization of Substance Use Disorders

An examination of history demonstrates a direct relationship between the criminalization of addiction and the racialization of substance use. One of the first laws against drug use in the United States was an ordinance passed in San Francisco in 1875 to ban the smoking of opium in opium dens, an activity thought to be associated with Chinese immigrants (Sacco 2014). The law was spurred by concerns that an activity that previously had been restricted to Chinese people was spreading to white people and morally bankrupting them (Sklansky 1995).

A century later, in the early 1980s, racialized depictions of the "dangerous Black crack cocaine fiend" began to rise in prominence. They were promoted by medical and legal authorities alike and echoed throughout the narratives of media and the chambers of governing bodies (Sklansky 1995). Medical authorities emphatically stated in a report to Congress that "cocaine is often the direct incentive to the crime of rape by Negroes of the South" (Sklansky 1995, p. 1292). These portrayals, in contrast to more favorable depictions of white users of powder cocaine, directly fueled differential federal drug sentencing guidelines. These guidelines, contained in the Anti-Drug Abuse Act of 1986, mandated penalties for crack cocaine–related fines that were 100 times harsher than penalties for powder cocaine–related crimes (Bailey et al. 2017). Although this discrepancy was lessened with the Fair Sentencing Act of 2010, it was not eliminated.

Early criminalization of cannabis was also largely rooted in racialized portrayals—this time of crazed Black and Mexican marijuana users (Bender 2016). In the early 1900s, it was asserted on the floor of the Texas Senate that "Mexicans are crazy, and this [marijuana] is what makes them crazy" (Bender 2016, p. 3). In the South, marijuana was portrayed as prompting murder, rape, and the seduction of white girls by Black men (Bender 2016). The 1936 exploitative film *Reefer Madness* furthered these racialized portrayals and coincided with widespread state bans of cannabis, followed by the federal Marijuana Tax Act of 1937 and marijuana's designation as an illegal, Schedule 1 drug (Bender 2016).

Notably, recent waves of decriminalization and legalization of marijuana have occurred not because of increased safety of cannabis but rather in light of its vast usage by white people, coinciding with more race-neutral public portrayals (Bender 2016). In fact, this decriminalization dovetails with an era of ever-increasing potency of cannabis on the market. Additionally, a growing body of scientific literature reflects more conclusive evidence of considerable negative health effects of cannabis, including the fact that it significantly accelerates the onset of psychotic illness in vulnerable individuals during years of crucial brain development (McGrath et al. 2010; National Institute on Drug Abuse 2020).

We need not wonder about what decriminalizing substance use in the United States might look like. In 2001, after extensive research and study, Portugal implemented full-scale decriminalization of the acquisition and possession of all "narcotics and psychotropic substances" for personal consumption by adults. Since this policy shift, lifetime prevalence rates of substance use have decreased for adolescents, although there have been slight increases in substance use for adults (Greenwald 2009). Rates of use of specific drug categories, including heroin, have decreased over time. Furthermore, rates of substance use in Portugal are among the lowest in all of the European Union. Most importantly, since decriminalization, there has been a significant decrease in newly reported cases of HIV, other sexually transmitted diseases, and drug-related deaths (Greenwald 2009). These positive outcomes make perfect sense: decriminalization allowed citizens of Portugal to seek treatment without fear of prosecution, and resources devoted to treatment in carceral settings were able to be reallocated toward community substance use disorder treatment programs. The United States, however, continues in the vein of punitive responses, an approach that intensified with the notorious "War on Drugs."

The War on Drug Users

Widespread prejudiced narratives about substance use disorders, variably supported by scientists but not usually supported by science, catalyzed the War on Drugs. Although this series of tough-on-crime policies initiated in the 1970s and 1980s did not refer to race directly, the policies disproportionately targeted people of color (Bailey et al. 2017). New York State's Rockefeller Drug Laws are one example. Enacted in 1973 under then-governor Nelson Rockefeller, these laws resulted in sentences for possession and sales of small quantities of drugs that were equal to or worse than sentences for many violent crimes, including rape, assault, and manslaughter (Drucker 2011). Importantly, sentence lengths were determined not by a jury but by mandatory sentencing policies that calculated prison sentences on the basis of weight and type of drug, as well as the defendant's criminal history (Drucker 2011).

By the late 1980s, at the peak of the crack cocaine epidemic, prisoners incarcerated in New York because of Rockefeller Drug Laws represented one-third of the entire prison population. In fact, people incarcerated under Rockefeller Drug Laws represented an increase of 1,733% from 1973 to 2001 (Drucker 2011). Nationwide, the war on drugs effectively fueled hyperincarceration, which in turn amplified the impact of other interlocking systems of structural racism, such as by differentially banning individuals from public housing and employment; restricting access to health care, voting, student loans, and the Supplemental Nutrition Assistance Program (SNAP); and removing parental rights, even after very short incarcerations (Bender 2016; Drucker 2011).

The literature is replete with debate on what the cocaine epidemic was or was not; however, critical examination reveals complicity between mass media, law enforcement, and politicians in circumscribing deviancy within the bodies of crack mothers and crack babies. Although the characterization of crack babies was more mythical than medical, this depiction persisted, and with significant consequences. It heightened the national outcry against crack cocaine and was employed to rationalize the War on Drugs despite the fact that a systematic review of the health effects on adolescents with in utero cocaine exposure found no consistent, statistically significant connection between cocaine exposure and poor health outcomes. Rather, differences in health outcomes were more clearly attributable to exposure to violence, trauma, and poverty—all conditions worsened by the structural violence enacted by the carceral system (Buckingham-Howes et al. 2013).

Although structural racism is pervasive throughout the carceral system, racial disproportionality in criminal sentencing is most pronounced in drug charges and is worst in cases of low-level drug offenses (Barnes and Kingsnorth 1996; Drucker 2011). In War on Drugs policies, explicitly racist language was not necessary for demonstrably racist impact. Rather, structural racism was mediated by many indirect factors highly susceptible to bias, such as selective enforcement by law enforcement officers and prosecutors, differential policing of neighborhoods, disparate penalty structures for different drugs, and discretionary or subjective assessment of intention to sell (Barnes and Kingsnorth 1996).

For example, under California law in the 1980s, possession of marijuana or methamphetamine (at that time used more prominently by white people) could be reduced to misdemeanors (Barnes and Kingsnorth 1996). In contrast, possession of cocaine or heroin (at that time used more prominently by people of color) could not be dropped to misdemeanors, warranted longer prison sentences, and were often treated more harshly than the *sale* of methamphetamine or marijuana (Barnes and Kingsnorth 1996). This differential legal treatment by drug type neither tracked with a scientific understanding of addiction nor aligned with the concept of relative harm. In fact, when compared with cocaine, methamphetamine has a much longer duration of action and more serious health effects, including an increase in the likelihood of psychosis (National Institute on Drug Abuse 2019).

As noted by Michelle Alexander (2010) in *The New Jim Crow*, some white Americans have been a form of collateral damage in the War on Drugs. For example, in more recent years, the media has often characterized methamphetamine as a drug used by poor, white, and rural people, and at the same time, the substance has been associated in the mind of the public with increased criminal activity. Policy responses have focused on law enforcement measures and supply chain legislation. These efforts have largely failed to drastically reduce the illegal production and ingestion of methamphetamine over time. The sensationalized media coverage of crystal meth use influenced the public and lawmakers, who then employed failed War on Drugs tactics. These included the aggressive arrest and incarceration of low-level drug offenders and subsequent postincarceration barriers to employment, voting, and obtaining public assistance.

These approaches amplify the marginalization of people who use crystal meth, particularly those in rural communities, and thereby bolster the narrative of their being irredeemable. As is the case for poor, urban Black people with substance use disorders, the primary barriers to treatment and recovery for people with methamphetamine use disorders are structural. Rurality presents a geographic barrier to care because local mental health care options may not treat methamphetamine use disorders or may not exist at all, and treatment in suburban or urban centers may be inaccessible because of transportation limitations. Although just under 20% of the U.S. population resides in rural counties, only 14% of outpatient substance use disorder treatment facilities are located in rural areas (U.S. Census Bureau 2016; Young et al. 2015). Additional geographically mediated inequities include limited family involvement due to distance, low numbers of health professionals who treat substance use disorders in rural settings, and inadequate access to peer support groups (Young et al. 2015). Another unmet need of the rural population results from the lack of integrated care that includes social services to support recovery efforts (Pringle et al. 2006).

Increased involvement of the child welfare system is an added downstream effect from the response to crack cocaine and rural methamphetamine use. For instance, when parents make and/or use crystal meth, the concerns for children include exposure to and risk for ingestion of toxic chemicals, the hazard posed by potentially explosive lab ingredients, and likely parental neglect while engaging in illicit use. These issues are certainly worthy of attention and appropriate interventions; however, this punitive carceral system–mediated approach has the collateral consequence of destabilizing families and undermining meaningful connection, a key element of recovery. For example, in California, adults caught manufacturing methamphetamine in the presence of children can be sentenced to prison. Although it is true that the immediate safety of these children must be secured in such circumstances, their chances for long-term security are better if their parents can access effective treatment and the children's number of placements can be minimized. The effects of parental incarceration on families are complex, and, predictably, the limitations imposed by incarceration impede parents' abilities to meet family reunification timelines and reunification plan requirements (Johnson and Waldfogel 2002). The Adoption Assistance and Child Welfare Act of 1980 and the Adoption and Safe Families Act of 1997 require states to file a petition to revoke parental rights after children have been in state care for 15 of the last 22 months. When these laws are coupled with lengthier methamphetamine sentences, reunification is precluded by structural barriers rather than parental disinterest or lack of commitment to recovery (Johnson and Waldfogel 2002).

Cocaine and Opioids: Similarities and Differences

The cocaine and opioid epidemics are strikingly dissimilar in public opinion and policy approaches; however, they are indistinguishable in their fidelity to the biopsychosocial etiologies of substance use disorders. Childhood trauma is one of the greatest risk factors for the development of substance use disorders in both women and men, illustrating the importance of understanding gene-environment interactions in the formulation of a drug epidemic (Giordano et al. 2016). It is also widely appreciated that human suffering and emotional pain can be among the key drivers of substance use, as well as of untreated or undertreated psychiatric disorders such as depression, anxiety, psychotic disorders, and impulse-control disorders, among others. Social determinants of poor health, such as unemployment and housing instability, are commonly elicited in the narrative histories of persons with substance use disorders. It is no coincidence that the cocaine and opioid epidemics both occurred in the context of economic downturns, historic job losses, and the increased availability of an addictive substance in their respective communities.

As highlighted throughout this chapter, public discourse is framed by media representations shaped by racism and classism. During the same era as the crack baby myth, mothers addicted to heroin had long been provided government-sanctioned methadone treatment as part of a medicalized response to prenatal exposures. Additionally, the sheer volume of media coverage for the opioid epidemic communicates the unique importance of the most commonly affected demographic, despite data supporting the need for a commensurate focus on cocaine, given the comparable health, social, and economic impacts (Shiels et al. 2018). Currently, one of the most striking dissimilarities is the quantity of media attention garnered by these two substances—there is a glaring disparity in coverage illuminating the rates of Black deaths from cocaine overdoses, even though they are commensurate with the rates of white deaths from opioids (Shiels et al. 2018).

Taken together, the intentional omission of biopsychosocial etiologies from the discourses of the crack cocaine epidemic and the lack of attention paid to Black deaths represent the devaluation of Black bodies as expendable casualties of the War on Drugs. The current foci of primary care, addiction medicine, and psychiatry rest squarely on the opioid epidemic, namely, prioritizing prescription drug misuse—rather than heroin use—at the expense of other ongoing epidemics. Despite exacting tolls on nonwhite and non-middle-class communities from other substance use disorders, billions of tax dollars have been directed to federal, state, and local programs earmarked to create a continuum of care *specifically* for opioid users.

Conclusion

The ramifications of social injustice in the societal response to and treatment of substance use disorders are profound, resulting in decades of devastation to individuals, families, and communities and compounding the oppression of already marginalized groups. Guided by an understanding of the scientific legitimacy of substance use disorders and the grievous public health impacts of criminalizing addiction, mental health professionals have the opportunity—and the responsibility—to shift public perception and, in turn, to shape policy and law. Mental health professionals can also lead by example, by reexamining their own clinical procedures and administrative policies and carefully searching for and eliminating barriers to accessing effective substance use disorder treatments. Such an apparent, unanimous affirmation of substance use disorders as a health issue, regardless of drug type or user demographic, would serve as an antidote to the structural violence enacted on individuals with substance use disorders, their families, and their communities.

Questions for Self-Reflection

1. Which drugs do I most associate with dangerousness and criminality? Are these associations rooted in medical knowledge or in stigma and bias?
2. What value judgments do I place on my patients with substance use disorders? What assumptions do I make about their character and their morals?
3. How does my practice or clinical setting address or perpetuate inequities in the treatment of different people with substance use disorders by drug? By race or by class?

References

Alexander M: The New Jim Crow: Mass Incarceration in the Age of Colorblindness. New York, New Press, 2010

American Psychiatric Association: Diagnostic and Statistical Manual of Mental Disorders, 4th Edition. Washington, DC, American Psychiatric Association, 1994

Appel O, Stephens D, Shadravan S, et al: Differential incarceration by race-ethnicity and mental health service status in the Los Angeles County jail system. Psychiatr Serv 71(8):843–846, 2020 Epub ahead of print

Bailey Z, Krieger N, Agénor M, et al: Structural racism and health inequities in the USA: evidence and interventions. Lancet 389:1453–1463, 2017

Barnes CW, Kingsnorth R: Race, drug, and criminal sentencing: hidden effects of the criminal law. J Crim Justice 24:39–55, 1996

Belenko S, Hiller M, Hamilton L: Treating substance use disorders in the criminal justice system. Curr Psychiatry Rep 15:414, 2013

Bender SW: The colors of cannabis: race and marijuana. UC Davis Law Rev 50:689–706, 2016

Buckingham-Howes S, Berger SS, Scaletti LA, Black MM: Systematic review of prenatal cocaine exposure and adolescent development. Pediatrics 131:e1917–e1936, 2013

Drucker E: A Plague of Prisons: The Epidemiology of Mass Incarceration in America. New York, New Press, 2011

Eversman MH, Bird JDP: Moral panic and social justice: a guide for analyzing social problems. Social Work 62:29–36, 2017

Giordano AL, Prosek EA, Stamman J, et al: Addressing trauma in substance abuse treatment. J Alcohol Drug Educ 60:55–71, 2016

Greenwald G: Drug Decriminalization in Portugal: Lessons for Creating Fair and Successful Drug Policies. Washington, DC, Cato Institute, 2009

Johnson E, Waldfogel J: Parental incarceration: recent trends and implications for child welfare. Soc Serv Rev 76:460–479, 2002

Link BG, Phelan JC: Conceptualizing stigma. Annu Rev Sociol 27:363–385, 2001

Logan E: The wrong race, committing crime, doing drugs, and maladjusted for motherhood: the nation's fury over "crack babies." Soc Justice 26:115–138, 1999

McGrath J, Welham J, Scott J, et al: Association between cannabis use and psychosis-related outcomes using sibling pair analysis in a cohort of young adults. Arch Gen Psychiatry 67:440–447, 2010

McLellan AT, Lewis DC, O'Brien CP, Kleber HD: Drug dependence, a chronic medical illness: implications for treatment, insurance, and outcomes evaluation. JAMA 284:1689–1695, 2000

McNeely J, Kumar PC, Rieckmann T, et al: Barriers and facilitators affecting the implementation of substance use screening in primary care clinics: a qualitative study of patients, providers, and staff. Addict Sci Clin Pract 13:8, 2018

National Institute on Drug Abuse: Methamphetamine: Research Report Series. Washington, DC, National Institute on Drug Abuse, October 2019. Available at: www.drugabuse.gov/publications/research-reports/methamphetamine/overview. Accessed May 4, 2020.

National Institute on Drug Abuse: Marijuana: Research Report Series. Washington, DC, National Institute on Drug Abuse, April 2020. Available at: www.drugabuse.gov/publications/research-reports/marijuana/letter-director. Accessed May 4, 2020.

Netherland J, Hansen HB: The war on drugs that wasn't: wasted whiteness, "dirty doctors," and race in media coverage of prescription opioid misuse. Cult Med Psychiatry 40:664–686, 2016

Office of the Surgeon General: Facing Addiction in America: The Surgeon General's Report on Alcohol, Drugs, and Health. Washington, DC, U.S. Department of Health and Human Services, 2016

Pringle J, Emptage N, Hubbard R: Unmet needs for comprehensive services in outpatient addiction treatment. J Subst Abuse Treat 30:183–189, 2006

Roberts NP, Roberts PA, Jones N, Bisson JI: Psychological interventions for post-traumatic stress disorder and comorbid substance use disorder: a systematic review and meta-analysis. Clin Psychol Rev 38:25–38, 2015

Sacco LN: Drug Enforcement in the United States: History, Policy, and Trends. Washington, DC, Congressional Research Service, 2014

Shiels MS, Freedman ND, Thomas D, Berrington de Gonzalez A: Trends in U.S. drug overdose deaths in non-Hispanic black, Hispanic, and non-Hispanic white persons, 2000–2015. Ann Intern Med 168:453–455, 2018

Sklansky D: Cocaine, race, and equal protection. Stanford Law Rev 47:1283–1322, 1995

Tsai AC, Kiang MV, Barnett ML, et al: Stigma as a fundamental hindrance to the United States opioid overdose crisis response. PLoS Med 16:e1002969, 2019

U.S. Census Bureau: Measuring America: Our Changing Landscape. Suitland, MD, U.S. Census Bureau, December 8, 2016. Available at: www.census.gov/content/dam/Census/library/visualizations/2016/comm/acs-rural-urban.pdf. Accessed May 10, 2020.

van Boekel LC, Brouwers EP, van Weeghel J, Garretsen HF: Stigma among health professionals towards patients with substance use disorders and its consequences for healthcare delivery: systematic review. Drug Alcohol Depend 131:23–35, 2013

Yang LH, Wong LY, Grivel MM, Hasin DS: Stigma and substance use disorders: an international phenomenon. Curr Opin Psychiatry 30:378–388, 2017

Young LB, Grant KM, Tyler KA: Community-level barriers to recovery for substance-dependent rural residents. J Soc Work Pract Addict 15:307–326, 2015

CHAPTER 11

Social Injustice and Schizophrenia

Khalima A. Bolden, Ph.D.
Poh Choo How, M.D., Ph.D.
Swati Rao, M.D.
Deidre M. Anglin, Ph.D.

Schizophrenia is a rare, chronic, and highly stigmatized mental illness that has evolved in its conceptualization along the fault lines of sociopolitical movements of the past century. Racial and political currents underlie the diagnosis, assessment, and treatment of schizophrenia, leading to significant mental health inequities. Currently, an accepted theoretical model for psychosis risk is the vulnerability-stress model, which hypothesizes that interactions between certain biological vulnerabilities (e.g., genetic predisposition, neurophysiological dysregulation) and environmental stressors (e.g., perinatal issues, adverse experiences, substance misuse) lead to the emergence of psychosis symptoms (Nuechterlein and Dawson 1984). However, the theorized origins of schizophrenia are highly sensitive to change over time.

In this chapter, we explore the history and evolution of the diagnosis of schizophrenia and ways in which the disorder has been weaponized to suppress Black communities. We discuss how generations of historical trauma coupled with ongoing traumatization increase the risk of the development of psychosis and how the social drift theory of schizophrenia has hindered the recovery of individuals and communities affected by psychosis by perpetuating health and socioeconomic disparities in disadvantaged communities.

Schizophrenia: The History of a Diagnosis

What is recognized today as schizophrenia was first characterized by Emil Kraepelin early in the twentieth century (Thomas 2001). He used the term *dementia praecox* to describe the premature appearance of cognitive symptoms in young patients seemingly suffering from a progressive neurodegenerative disease. Later, the word *schizophrenia* was coined by Eugen Bleuler in 1911, from the Greek words *schizein*, indicating splitting, and *phren*, to denote the psyche. In the first edition of DSM (American Psychiatric Association 1952), schizophrenia was conceptualized as a disease of personality disintegration, leading to disturbances in thinking, mood, and behaviors such as retreating from reality and regression. Thus, in its infancy, in a departure from the original conceptualization of a neurobiological process, schizophrenia was considered a disorder impacting people with *sensitive dispositions* and *weaker minds and personalities* who were susceptible to this splitting of the psyche.

In the 1950s, Kurt Schneider proposed a greater focus on positive symptoms such as hallucinations and delusions (i.e., first-rank symptoms) in the diagnosis of schizophrenia. In the same decade, the discovery of antipsychotics (which emerged from research on tranquilizers) and their use in the treatment of schizophrenia contributed to a shift in the conceptualization of schizophrenia from a disease of a "weak mind" to one of "crazy, unpredictable, and dangerous" behavior, at least in the public mind (Katschnig 2018). This shift in perception paralleled the growing civil rights movements of the 1960s. When DSM-II was published in 1968, its overview of schizophrenia placed greater emphasis on hallucinations and delusions and on inappropriate emotional responsiveness, loss of empathy with others, and bizarre behaviors (American Psychiatric Association 1968).

By the time DSM-III was published in 1980 (American Psychiatric Association 1980), Schneider's first-rank symptoms were cemented into the criteria for schizophrenia, and in DSM-III-R, subtypes of schizophrenia were introduced, including the paranoid subtype, for which the description included "unfocused anxiety, anger, argumentativeness, and violence"

(American Psychiatric Association 1987). These descriptions were removed in DSM-5 (American Psychiatric Association 2013) because they did not adequately reflect the heterogeneity of schizophrenia. Although the first edition of DSM emphasized the degree of functional impairment in the diagnostic criteria, later versions stressed the presence of specific symptoms, as reflected in DSM-5 (Box 11–1).

Box 11–1. DSM-5 Criteria for Schizophrenia

A. Two (or more) of the following, each present for a significant portion of time during a 1-month period (or less if successfully treated). At least one of these must be (1), (2), or (3):

   1. Delusions.
   2. Hallucinations.
   3. Disorganized speech (e.g., frequent derailment or incoherence).
   4. Grossly disorganized or catatonic behavior.
   5. Negative symptoms (i.e., diminished emotional expression or avolition).

B. For a significant portion of the time since the onset of the disturbance, level of functioning in one or more major areas, such as work, interpersonal relations, or self-care, is markedly below the level achieved prior to the onset (or when the onset is in childhood or adolescence, there is failure to achieve expected level of interpersonal, academic, or occupational functioning).

C. Continuous signs of the disturbance persist for at least 6 months. This 6-month period must include at least 1 month of symptoms (or less if successfully treated) that meet Criterion A (i.e., active-phase symptoms) and may include periods of prodromal or residual symptoms. During these prodromal or residual periods, the signs of the disturbance may be manifested by only negative symptoms or by two or more symptoms listed in Criterion A present in an attenuated form (e.g., odd beliefs, unusual perceptual experiences).

D. Schizoaffective disorder and depressive or bipolar disorder with psychotic features have been ruled out because either 1) no major depressive or manic episodes have occurred concurrently with the active-phase symptoms, or 2) if mood episodes have occurred during active-phase symptoms, they have been present for a minority of the total duration of the active and residual periods of the illness.

E. The disturbance is not attributable to the physiological effects of a substance (e.g., a drug of abuse, a medication) or another medical condition.

F. If there is a history of autism spectrum disorder or a communication disorder of childhood onset, the additional diagnosis of schizophrenia is made only if prominent delusions or hallucinations, in addition to the other required symptoms of schizophrenia, are also present for at least 1 month (or less if successfully treated).

Specify if:

The following course specifiers are only to be used after a 1-year duration of the disorder and if they are not in contradiction to the diagnostic course criteria.

First episode, currently in acute episode: First manifestation of the disorder meeting the defining diagnostic symptom and time criteria. An *acute episode* is a time period in which the symptom criteria are fulfilled.

First episode, currently in partial remission: *Partial remission* is a period of time during which an improvement after a previous episode is maintained and in which the defining criteria of the disorder are only partially fulfilled.

First episode, currently in full remission: *Full remission* is a period of time after a previous episode during which no disorder-specific symptoms are present.

Multiple episodes, currently in acute episode: Multiple episodes may be determined after a minimum of two episodes (i.e., after a first episode, a remission and a minimum of one relapse).

Multiple episodes, currently in partial remission

Multiple episodes, currently in full remission

Continuous: Symptoms fulfilling the diagnostic symptom criteria of the disorder are remaining for the majority of the illness course, with subthreshold symptom periods being very brief relative to the overall course.

Unspecified

Specify if:

With catatonia (refer to the criteria for catatonia associated with another mental disorder, pp. 119–120, for definition).

Coding note: Use additional code 293.89 (F06.1) catatonia associated with schizophrenia to indicate the presence of the comorbid catatonia.

Specify current severity:

Severity is rated by a quantitative assessment of the primary symptoms of psychosis, including delusions, hallucinations, disorganized speech, abnormal psychomotor behavior, and negative symptoms. Each of these symptoms may be rated for its current severity (most severe in the last 7 days) on a 5-point scale ranging from 0 (not present) to 4 (present and severe). (See Clinician-Rated Dimensions of Psychosis Symptom Severity in the chapter "Assessment Measures.")

Note: Diagnosis of schizophrenia can be made without using this severity specifier.

As previously alluded to, the history and evolution of the diagnostic criteria for schizophrenia did not occur in isolation from the sociopolitical climate of the United States. Changes in the diagnostic criteria were intimately linked with the media's portrayal of the disease, the demographics of individuals who were diagnosed with schizophrenia, and the treatment they received.

Racial Bias in the Diagnosis and Treatment of Schizophrenia

In his groundbreaking book *The Protest Psychosis: How Schizophrenia Became a Black Disease*, Jonathan Metzl (2010) tracked the ways the public and scientific understanding of schizophrenia changed in response to sociopolitical changes over time through an examination of thousands of records of patients who received the diagnosis at the Ionia State Hospital in Michigan from the 1940s until its closure in the late 1970s. Before the early 1960s, patients at Ionia were nonviolent white male offenders and white women. Psychiatrists' assessments of symptoms of mental illness in the women included the following: "wasn't able to take care of her family as she should," "can't do her housework," and "talked too loudly and embarrassed her husband" (Metzl 2010, p. 10). In other words, women who were unable to meet rigid gendered expectations or who exhibited resistance to socially acceptable behavior were pathologized as having weak, fractured minds and personalities and were diagnosed with schizophrenia. Metzl hypothesized about one patient in particular: "Perhaps [she] rebelled against a patriarchal system, and a patriarchal diagnosis, that allowed white male doctors and her white male husband to be the arbiters of her mental health.... [H]owever, the most important aspect...is that [her] defiance was interpreted as a symptom but not as a threat" (Metzl 2010, p. 44).

Accordingly, the treatment of schizophrenia in these women focused on improving their adherence to their roles as wives and mothers. Therapeutic interventions included sewing, playing music, making pottery, and cooking. Life in the hospital closely mimicked life outside the hospital, including interactions with the public through regular community outings. Despite these patients' classification as "criminally insane," both the community and mental health professionals at Ionia felt safe and unthreatened in their interactions with these patients. Journal and media articles from the era described people with schizophrenia as docile and tame, and advertisements for medication commonly portrayed placid, usually white women calmly reading or knitting. At the time, common conceptualizations of schizophrenia did not include symptoms of paranoia, aggression, or hostility (Metzl 2010). Instead, schizophrenia was conceptualized as a disease resulting from early-life psychological trauma, often committed at the hands of a schizophrenogenic mother (Hartwell 1996).

In the 1960s, the understanding of schizophrenia shifted from a disease affecting the "weak psyches" of women to a behavioral disease of dangerous, rage-filled men in the setting of political and social discord stirred by the civil rights movement (Metzl 2010). The phrase *protest psychosis* was coined by Bromberg and Simon (1968) to describe a reactive psychosis arising in Black males as a result of "the stress of asserting civil rights in the United States" (p. 155). Bromberg and Simon described symptoms that they likened to schizophrenia, paranoid type, but also identified as being more distinctive, including hallucinations of African themes, adoption of Islamic doctrine, and promotion of antiwhite mindsets. Ultimately, they hypothesized that this reactive psychosis "joins with a racial unconscious identification to attack the traditional values established by white humanity" (Bromberg and Simon 1968, p. 156). At the time, researchers claimed that Black psychiatric patients had higher measures of hostility than white psychiatric patients, stemming from "delusional beliefs that their civil rights were being compromised or violated" (Metzl 2010, p. 101; Raskin et al. 1975).

Absent from this discussion of psychosis was the acknowledgment that the stress experienced by Black people derived from mistreatment by white society over several centuries rather than from asserting their civil rights. The academic tone of the various authors does not hide their astonishment that anyone would disagree with the obvious superiority of the white race over other races. This shift in the construction of schizophrenia as a disease of aggression and hostility in young Black men did not occur as a coincidence during the civil rights era but was the direct response of white psychiatrists to the demand for equal treatment by Black Americans. Large-scale pathologizing of the tenets of the civil rights movement by equating these ideas with paranoid delusions allowed certain sectors of society a mechanism for removing threats to the status quo in the name of safety and mental health. This was reflected in the clinical data at Ionia State Hospital, where, by the mid-1970s, the overwhelming majority of patients diagnosed with schizophrenia were Black men (Metzl 2010).

The shift in the diagnostic criteria and the demographics of individuals diagnosed with schizophrenia catalyzed a change in treatment approaches. As more young Black men were being diagnosed with schizophrenia, the lines between the illness, violence, and criminal behavior became blurred. Psychiatric asylums became increasingly populated by Black men diagnosed with schizophrenia, and psychiatrists began documenting perceived hostility, aggression, and belligerence, establishing an increased need for seclusion and restraints to control these patients (Metzl 2010). Additional security was added to psychiatric asylums because "dangerous" patients had to be locked up and secured—isolated from the public. Unsurprisingly, asylums such as Ionia State Hospital shifted from idyllic farmland settings to maximum-security facilities. Concurrently, the shift in the conceptualization of schizophrenia as a biological disease rather than a psychological reaction to trauma reflected a belief in the biological inferiority of non-Europeans and that this biological imbalance required treatment with newly developed biochemical therapies. The advertisements for these pharmaceutical agents portrayed patients as dangerous individuals who needed to be subdued and tranquilized (Metzl 2010).

The paranoid subtype of schizophrenia, although only officially introduced in DSM in the 1980s, has its roots in protest psychosis. In the 1980s and 1990s, Black men were diagnosed with paranoid schizophrenia at a rate five to seven times that of white men (Metzl 2010). Although psychiatrists today may be shocked by the blatant racist and sexist language used by psychiatrists of prior generations, many of these disturbing biases persist today. Psychiatrists continue to overdiagnose schizophrenia and paranoia and underdiagnose mood disorders in Black men compared with white men (Gara et al. 2019; Strakowski et al. 2003). Furthermore, psychiatrists tend to overestimate violence in Black patients while underestimating violence in white patients (Hicks 2004). As a result of these biases, Black patients are more likely to be hospitalized involuntarily, to be administered higher doses of antipsychotics, to be administered medications against their will, and to be secluded and restrained (Rost et al. 2011). Such data may be regarded as unfortunate and unintended consequences of the actions of a prior, misguided generation, especially when considering that this history is usually omitted from psychiatric training and education. However, a thorough inspection of this history reveals that these current biased trends are the purposeful result of meticulously created diagnostic structures from not so long ago.

Trauma and Schizophrenia

It would be easy to dismiss the blatant racism of psychiatrists in the 1960s as a thing of the past; however, this racism played an integral role in shaping the institutional structure, procedures, and policies of psychiatric practice today. This process did not merely begin in the twentieth century with the civil rights movement. Historical trauma in Black communities has contributed to both an increased vulnerability to psychosis and the misdiagnosis of schizophrenia in these populations. Additionally, as a by-product of social drift theory, Black populations have been historically excluded from effective treatment and recovery from schizophrenia.

Historical trauma is the "cumulative emotional and psychological wounding, over the lifespan and across generations, emanating from massive group trauma experiences" (Brave Heart 2003, p. 7). The following are the four basic assumptions of historical trauma theory (Sotero 2006):

1. Mass trauma is intentionally inflicted on the target population.
2. Trauma is not a singular event but a continuous and prolonged exposure.
3. Traumatic events resound throughout the population, creating a collective experience.
4. The developmental trajectory of the targeted population is irrevocably altered, resulting in inequities that persist through generations.

Much of the research on historical trauma has examined Jewish communities and Holocaust survivors and, more recently, Japanese American and Native American marginalization and enclosure in the United States. This work has helped to elucidate that this type of trauma is not a result of a single event but rather a result of deep psychological harm arising from a wide array of events and experiences that interact with development over time and exist in an intergenerational cultural context (Danzer et al. 2016).

Although few studies have specifically examined historical trauma in Black communities, any basic understanding of U.S. history identifies repeated, prolonged, and massive group traumas inflicted on Black Americans across generations, including chattel slavery, Jim Crow laws enforcing racial segregation, overpolicing of Black communities, mass incarceration, and multiple instances (both in the past and more recently) of inhumane and unethical medical experimentation. Not only are Black people vulnerable to being violently traumatized, but there is a shared vulnerability within Black communities based on historical and present-day events where day-to-day experiences of racism, discrimination, microaggressions, and macroaggressions touch on the collective trauma carried over generations.

Groups touched by historical trauma are collectively more vulnerable to a host of mental health issues, including PTSD and psychosis (Hardy and Mueser 2017; Sotero 2006). Evidence for a link between trauma and psychosis is well established in the case of adverse childhood experiences and psychotic symptoms (Powers et al. 2016). Current theories linking trauma and psychosis posit the development of psychotic symptoms such as hallucinations as a dimension of PTSD (Hardy and Mueser 2017). At the same time, symptoms of both PTSD and trauma-related psychosis are often used to support a diagnosis of schizophrenia and other psychotic disorders. Symptoms such as hypervigilance in PTSD may be interpreted as paranoia, and hallucinations related to trauma may be used to substantiate the diagnosis of a psychotic disorder. Additionally, legitimate mistrust of government, legal, and medical institutions as a result of structural violence perpetrated by these institutions against Black communities often manifests as the inclination to avoid doctors or refuse prescribed medications, a reaction that mental health professionals may interpret as suspiciousness and paranoia (LaVeist et al. 2000). Hence, as a sequela of historical trauma, members of Black communities are more vulnerable to the development of psychotic symptoms and simultaneously to the misdiagnosis of a psychotic disorder if their symptoms are not viewed through the lens of historical (and current) trauma.

Therefore, the evaluation of psychotic symptoms in populations with historical trauma exposure calls for a cultural humility approach. Cultural humility emphasizes redressing the power imbalance between a provider and a patient. This approach acknowledges that patients are the experts of their own lived experiences and that the knowledge and context provided by patients are valued, important information (Tervalon and Murray-Garcia 1998). It also calls for self-reflection and self-critique on the part of providers in understanding the limitations of their knowledge and training (e.g., taking into account the historical biases in the development of diagnostic criteria for schizophrenia).

Case Example

Andrew is a 25-year-old Black man who was referred to an outpatient mental health clinic for evaluation and treatment of a possible psychotic disorder. The referral requested psychological and psychiatric evaluations after recent issues at his firm. When Andrew initially presented for treatment, he reported that he was told he had to come to treatment because he was not getting along with coworkers he believed were racist and discriminating against him. He also shared that he had been experiencing feelings of isolation and social rejection. He expressed concerns that his coworkers were out to get him and that he sometimes felt that they were trying to prevent him from being successful at his work. When asked about his family history, he informed the clinician that his mother had a primary psychotic disorder. The evaluating psychologist administered a variety of self-report measures, including the Minnesota Multiphasic Personality Inventory–2 (MMPI-2), on which Andrew scored in the clinically elevated range on the Antisocial Behavior and Ideas of Persecution scales. Following this assessment, Andrew was diagnosed with unspecified schizophrenia spectrum and other psychotic disorder and was referred for further evaluation to a psychologist specializing in the treatment of early psychosis.

During his initial evaluation session with the psychologist, Andrew reported worrying about what his coworkers thought of him because they had to do a lot of team-based projects, which were awkward and uncomfortable. When asked why he believed his coworkers disliked him and why he felt they were discriminating against him, he related several incidents in which he suffered microaggressions as well as overt discriminatory statements. Andrew recounted that one of his coworkers told him, "You know you are only here because of affirmative action, right?" and another coworker implied that Andrew did not have to work as hard on their projects because, as the only Black man in the company, his job at the firm was secure. Andrew also discussed being suspicious of some of the people at his church and apartment complex. When asked why, he noted it was because he was a "Black man in the South," and he was not sure if he could trust people in the current political climate in the United States. He reported feeling suspicious of all white people but particularly of those he knew and had to work with or interact with closely because he believed that many white people are racist. Following this discussion, the psychologist administered a structured diagnostic interview that did not reveal any evidence of psychosis. However, Andrew did endorse increasing apathy and anhedonia, decreased appetite, hypersomnia, increased irritability, difficulty concentrating, and feelings of worthlessness. The psychologist diagnosed Andrew with major depressive disorder, and he was referred for treatment with an emphasis on systemic and interpersonal discrimination-associated stress.

On the basis of Andrew's thoughts about his coworkers, his family history, and the results of psychological testing, the initial evaluating clinician referred him for a specialized evaluation for psychosis. Andrew waited for this specialized assessment for several months and meanwhile was unable to work because he needed a doctor's note to clear him to return to work. The prolonged diagnostic evaluation process, which spanned 6 months, did not endear Andrew to the idea of ongoing treatment. Consistent with many mental health professionals (Gara et al. 2019), the referring clinician underemphasized Andrew's depressive symptoms and failed to appreciate the lasting impact of historical and current trauma in his life. Psychosis was placed at the top of the differential diagnosis not because the referring clinician was racist or incompetent but likely because of a misunderstanding of the context of Andrew's experiences at work coupled with a lack of clinician knowledge regarding the questionable diagnostic validity of standardized clinical assessments such as the MMPI-2.

Social Drift and Social Causation

Early research examining the relationship between socioeconomic factors and schizophrenia observed an increased incidence of schizophrenia among individuals from neighborhoods with high rates of poverty, socially disorganized residential areas, marital instability, and residential mobility (Faris and

Dunham 1939). To explain this finding, proponents of the *social drift hypothesis* postulated that psychotic patients tend to gradually undergo downward social mobility into economically deprived neighborhoods as a result of unemployment, a decline in cognitive functioning, and other social difficulties associated with experiencing psychotic symptoms (Goldberg and Morrison 1963). For most of the twentieth century—and, to a lesser extent, today—social drift has been widely accepted as a natural course of schizophrenia.

Reliance on social drift theory to explain the low socioeconomic status of patients with schizophrenia erases the important role of social factors in triggering psychosis (Jarvis 2007). Much of psychiatric research and training has focused primarily on the genetic inheritance of schizophrenia, in part because this perspective reaffirms societal biases about the biological inferiority of minority groups who are overrepresented in the diagnosis of schizophrenia. At the same time, research into social factors such as poverty, migration, and racial discrimination in the etiology of schizophrenia has been lacking. Instead, these factors are viewed as confounding variables that are statistically controlled to reveal the more significant trends in data. The lack of data in this realm also allows mental health professionals to ignore the larger role of structural inequities that contribute to the development of psychosis in marginalized, disenfranchised, and minoritized communities and absolves mental health professionals from taking action to address these inequities.

In contrast to the lack of research in the United States, various social causation interpretations have arisen out of Europe based on research into many adverse social and neighborhood factors, which have been shown to increase the risk of developing psychosis among the genetically vulnerable. The original data by Faris and Dunham (1939) already supported the causal role of social exclusion as a risk factor for schizophrenia, with the finding that Black people had higher rates of hospital admissions for psychosis only when they lived in neighborhoods where they were the minority of residents. In recent decades, research in Europe has connected social exclusion with an increased risk of psychotic disorders. For example, children from single-parent households had a higher risk of developing a psychotic disorder than did children from two-parent households only when they attended schools in which very few peers belonged to the same background (Zammit et al. 2010). Discrimination is also an independent risk factor for psychosis, and experiencing multiple forms of discrimination increases the risk of developing psychosis in a dose-dependent fashion (Stickley et al. 2019).

The *social defeat hypothesis* proposes a pathway through which chronic discrimination, adversity, and isolation can lead to psychosis. Animal models simulating social subordination and isolation suggest that chronic social defeat may increase the risk for schizophrenia through an increase in baseline dopaminergic activity (Cantor-Graae 2007). Positron emission tomography studies in humans with a high risk for developing mental illness show an increased dopamine response when a stressful task is combined with negative feedback (Selten et al. 2013).

Studies of social exclusion and social defeat highlight the importance of understanding an individual's social context rather than the individual's characteristics on their own. These studies implicate structural discrimination and inequity in the etiology of schizophrenia. These injustices pose bidirectional risks in the development of psychosis. Existing injustices themselves lead to a greater risk of developing psychosis. Once an individual has developed psychosis, injustices further limit access to evaluation, treatment, and the social change needed for any chance of recovery. This reciprocal causality is supported by research showing a higher rate of mental illness recovery in individuals with a higher socioeconomic status compared with those who are socioeconomically disadvantaged, as mediated through access to or use of health services (Sweeney et al. 2015).

Conclusion

Racial inequities in the diagnosis, assessment, and treatment of psychotic disorders are steeped in a long history of historical trauma and structural inequities experienced by Black Americans and other oppressed groups. Far from being objective measures, the diagnostic criteria for psychosis and schizophrenia have been influenced by societal forces that have weaponized these criteria to oppress and discriminate against populations that have dared to express a desire to fight against their oppression. Schizophrenia is a debilitating disease that is largely considered to be primarily biological. Unfortunately, throughout history, it is also an illness that has been conceptualized by some people to emphasize white male superiority. Thus, efforts to understand the contribution of trauma, oppression, and social injustice to the etiology of schizophrenia have been lacking. Dismantling the underlying structural inequalities contributing to the overdiagnosis and misdiagnosis of schizophrenia in Black men, coupled with a lack of resources for the effective treatment of psychosis, is imperative in addressing the inequities seen in the diagnosis and treatment of schizophrenia (Metzl and Hansen 2014).

Questions for Self-Reflection

1. What have I assumed were the causes of higher rates of diagnoses of schizophrenia in Black men?
2. How might my implicit biases impact the way I evaluate, diagnose, and treat Black men with psychotic symptoms?
3. How can I be more intentional about applying an equity lens to the diagnosis and treatment of psychotic and mood disorders in my patients?

References

American Psychiatric Association: Diagnostic and Statistical Manual of Mental Disorders. Washington, DC, American Psychiatric Association, 1952

American Psychiatric Association: Diagnostic and Statistical Manual of Mental Disorders, 2nd Edition. Washington, DC, American Psychiatric Association, 1968

American Psychiatric Association: Diagnostic and Statistical Manual of Mental Disorders, 3rd Edition. Washington, DC, American Psychiatric Association, 1980

American Psychiatric Association: Diagnostic and Statistical Manual of Mental Disorders, 3rd Edition, Revised. Washington, DC, American Psychiatric Association, 1987

American Psychiatric Association: Diagnostic and Statistical Manual of Mental Disorders, 5th Edition. Arlington, VA, American Psychiatric Association, 2013

Brave Heart MYH: The historical trauma response among natives and its relationship with substance abuse: a Lakota illustration. J Psychoactive Drugs 35:7–13, 2003

Bromberg W, Simon F: The protest psychosis: a special type of reactive psychosis. Arch Gen Psychiatry 19:155–160, 1968

Cantor-Graae E: The contribution of social factors to the development of schizophrenia: a review of recent findings. Can J Psychiatry 52:277–286, 2007

Danzer G, Rieger SM, Schubmehl S, Cort D: White psychologists and African Americans' historical trauma: implications for practice. J Aggress Maltreat Trauma 25:351–370, 2016

Faris RE, Dunham HW: Mental Disorders in Urban Areas: An Ecological Study of Schizophrenia and Other Psychoses. Chicago, IL, University of Chicago Press, 1939

Gara MA, Minsky S, Silverstein SM, Miskimen T, et al: A naturalistic study of racial disparities in diagnoses at an outpatient behavioral health clinic. Psychiatr Serv 70:130–134, 2019

Goldberg EM, Morrison SL: Schizophrenia and social class. Br J Psychiatry 109:785–802, 1963

Hardy KV, Mueser KT: Trauma, psychosis and posttraumatic stress disorder. Front Psychiatry 8:220, 2017

Hartwell CE: The schizophrenogenic mother concept in American psychiatry. Psychiatry 59:274–297, 1996

Hicks JW: Ethnicity, race, and forensic psychiatry: are we color-blind? J Am Acad Psychiatry Law 32:21–33, 2004

Jarvis GE: The social causes of psychosis in North American psychiatry: a review of a disappearing literature. Can J Psychiatry 52:287–294, 2007

Katschnig H: Psychiatry's contribution to the public stereotype of schizophrenia: historical considerations. J Eval Clin Pract 24:1093–1100, 2018

LaVeist TA, Nickerson KJ, Bowie JV: Attitudes about racism, medical mistrust, and satisfaction with care among African American and white cardiac patients. Med Care Res Rev 75:146–161, 2000

Metzl JM: The Protest Psychosis: How Schizophrenia Became a Black Disease. Boston, MA, Beacon, 2010

Metzl J, Hansen H: Structural competency: theorizing a new medical engagement with stigma and inequality. Soc Sci Med 103:126–133, 2014

Nuechterlein KH, Dawson ME: A heuristic vulnerability/stress model of schizophrenic episodes. Schizophr Bull 10:300–312, 1984

Powers A, Fani N, Cross D, et al: Childhood trauma, PTSD, and psychosis: findings from a highly traumatized, minority sample. Child Abuse Negl 58:111–118, 2016

Raskin A, Crook TH, Herman KD: Psychiatric history and symptom differences in black and white depressed patients. J Consult Clin Psychol 43:73–80, 1975

Rost K, Hsieh YP, Xu S, et al: Potential disparities in the management of schizophrenia in the United States. Psychiatr Serv 62:613–618, 2011

Selten JP, van der Ven E, Rutten BP, Cantor-Graae E: The social defeat hypothesis of schizophrenia: an update. Schizophr Bull 39:1180–1186, 2013

Sotero M: A conceptual model of historical trauma: implications for public health practice and research. J Health Dispar Res Pract 1:93–108, 2006

Stickley A, Oh H, Sumiyoshi T, et al: Perceived discrimination and psychotic experiences in the English general population. Eur Psychiatry 62:50–57, 2019

Strakowski SM, Keck PE, Arnold LM, et al: Ethnicity and diagnosis in patients with affective disorder. J Clin Psychiatry 64:747–754, 2003

Sweeney S, Air T, Zannettino L, Galletly C: Psychosis, socioeconomic disadvantage, and health service use in South Australia: findings from the Second Australian National Survey of Psychosis. Front Public Health 3:259, 2015

Tervalon M, Murray-Garcia J: Cultural humility versus cultural competence: a critical distinction in defining physician training outcomes in multicultural education. J Health Care Poor Underserved 9:117–125, 1998

Thomas AB: Evolution of diagnostic criteria in psychoses. Dialogues Clin Neurosci 3:257–263, 2001

Zammit S, Lewis G, Rasbash J, et al: Individuals, schools, and neighborhood: a multilevel longitudinal study of variation in incidence of psychotic disorders. Arch Gen Psychiatry 67:914–922, 2010

CHAPTER 12

Social Injustice and Personality Disorders

David Freedman, Ph.D.
George W. Woods, M.D., LFAPA

Suppose an adolescent has been exposed to lead, which results in cognitive deficits, disruptive behaviors in school, and subsequent criminal conduct, and is then referred by a juvenile justice case manager for an outpatient psychiatric evaluation. In a significant majority of instances, the lead exposure will not be known to the evaluating psychiatrist. What will be known are the disruptive and criminal behaviors that brought the adolescent into the assessment setting. What does the psychiatrist see when this adolescent comes in for an assessment? Often, the psychiatrist will observe someone who is unable to conform to the rules of school and engages in behaviors that most typically result in antisocial or borderline diagnostic labels, especially when the adolescent is a person of color or comes from a neighborhood of concentrated poverty. Diagnostically, does this adolescent have a personality disorder? A cognitive impairment secondary to lead exposure? A medical condition (lead poisoning) that requires treatment? The easy answer is all of the above, but that is an insufficient causal answer and a clinically inappropriate answer because it guides the psychiatrist to recommend the wrong treatment protocol. Core to the assessment will be the psychiatrist's implicit and explicit biases about the gender, race, and economic status of the adolescent. This adolescent, on the basis of these facts, does not have a characterological or personality disorder that manifests as criminal behavior; he or she has been exposed to a neurotoxin, and with appropriate treatment, the condition could potentially be remediated or resolved.

In this chapter, we address some of the issues related to how and why personality disorders are diagnosed, how bias affects the assessment process, and some of the consequences of labeling a person as personality disordered. After a brief review of the diagnostic criteria, we explore the significant problems in how personality disorders are conceptualized; briefly consider some of the reliability and validity issues raised by those faulty conceptualizations; and address how social inequity impacts the diagnosis of a personality disorder as well as how the diagnosis reinforces those inequities.

Defining Antisocial and Borderline Personality Disorders

DSM-5 (American Psychiatric Association 2013) defines a personality disorder as "an enduring pattern of inner experience and behavior that deviates markedly from the expectations of the individual's culture, is pervasive and inflexible, has an onset in adolescence or early adulthood, is stable over time, and leads to distress or impairment" (p. 645). This definition applies to the 10 personality disorders in DSM-5, which are grouped into three clusters. The focus of this chapter is on two of the Cluster B personality disorders: antisocial personality disorder (ASPD; Box 12–1) and borderline personality disorder (BPD; Box 12–2).

Prevalence rates of ASPD range from 0.2% in the general population to 70% in males with alcohol use disorders and inmates and higher among individuals affected by poverty and sociocultural factors (American Psychiatric Association 2013). DSM-5 states explicitly that ASPD "appears to be associated with low socioeconomic status and urban settings" (p. 662), and it is diagnosed much more often in men. The supposed association between race, class, gender, and ASPD is one central focus of this chapter. Prevalence rates of BPD range between 1.6% in the general population and 20% in psychiatric inpatient samples (American Psychiatric Association 2013). BPD is diagnosed overwhelmingly in women. It was added to the DSM-III nomenclature in 1980.

Box 12–1.   DSM-5 Criteria for Antisocial Personality Disorder

---

A. A pervasive pattern of disregard for and violation of the rights of others, occurring since age 15 years, as indicated by three (or more) of the following:

 1. Failure to conform to social norms with respect to lawful behaviors, as indicated by repeatedly performing acts that are grounds for arrest.
 2. Deceitfulness, as indicated by repeated lying, use of aliases, or conning others for personal profit or pleasure.
 3. Impulsivity or failure to plan ahead.
 4. Irritability and aggressiveness, as indicated by repeated physical fights or assaults.
 5. Reckless disregard for safety of self or others.
 6. Consistent irresponsibility, as indicated by repeated failure to sustain consistent work behavior or honor financial obligations.
 7. Lack of remorse, as indicated by being indifferent to or rationalizing having hurt, mistreated, or stolen from another.

B. The individual is at least age 18 years.
C. There is evidence of conduct disorder with onset before age 15 years.
D. The occurrence of antisocial behavior is not exclusively during the course of schizophrenia or bipolar disorder.

Source.   Reprinted from American Psychiatric Association: Diagnostic and Statistical Manual of Mental Disorders, 5th Edition. Arlington, VA, American Psychiatric Association, 2013, p. 659. Copyright © 2013 American Psychiatric Association. Used with permission.

DSM-5 also includes an alternative model of personality disorders in an appendix, with the suggestion that this model may eventually replace the current model. The alternative model locates people dimensionally along a spectrum such that everyone would have some amount of the symptoms, but a certain level of impairment is needed for a diagnosis. The model maintains the essential criteria for ASPD and BPD, but diagnosis requires impairment in personality functioning and pathological personality traits (American Psychiatric Association 2013). For an individual to be diagnosed with either ASPD or BPD, the alternative model requires moderate or greater impairment in identity, self-direction, empathy, and intimacy, along with pathological traits as defined for each disorder.

Box 12–2.   DSM-5 Criteria for Borderline Personality Disorder

---

A pervasive pattern of instability of interpersonal relationships, self-image, and affects, and marked impulsivity, beginning by early adulthood and present in a variety of contexts, as indicated by five (or more) of the following:

1. Frantic efforts to avoid real or imagined abandonment. (**Note:** Do not include suicidal or self-mutilating behavior covered in Criterion 5.)
2. A pattern of unstable and intense interpersonal relationships characterized by alternating between extremes of idealization and devaluation.
3. Identity disturbance: markedly and persistently unstable self-image or sense of self.
4. Impulsivity in at least two areas that are potentially self-damaging (e.g., spending, sex, substance abuse, reckless driving, binge eating). (**Note:** Do not include suicidal or self-mutilating behavior covered in Criterion 5.)
5. Recurrent suicidal behavior, gestures, or threats, or self-mutilating behavior.
6. Affective instability due to a marked reactivity of mood (e.g., intense episodic dysphoria, irritability, or anxiety usually lasting a few hours and only rarely more than a few days).
7. Chronic feelings of emptiness.
8. Inappropriate, intense anger or difficulty controlling anger (e.g., frequent displays of temper, constant anger, recurrent physical fights).
9. Transient, stress-related ideation or severe dissociative symptoms.

Source.   Reprinted from American Psychiatric Association: Diagnostic and Statistical Manual of Mental Disorders, 5th Edition. Arlington, VA, American Psychiatric Association, 2013, p. 659. Copyright © 2013 American Psychiatric Association. Used with permission.

Antisocial and Borderline Personality Disorders Are Neither Immutable Nor Stable Over Time

As defined, personality disorders begin early in life and are fixed, immutable characteristics that persist across the life span. Despite this assertion, the longitudinal research on personality disorders does not support this claim. First, taking the criteria at face value, the characteristics that make up personality disorders are not fixed and immutable over the life span, which raises doubt as to the validity of the concept. For instance, in a population-based Norwegian twin study in which 2,270 participants with ASPD and 2,269 participants with BPD were assessed first at a mean age of 28 years and then again at a mean age of 38 years, the mean number of criteria for ASPD fell from 0.42 to 0.25 (a 40% decline) and for BPD from 0.99 to 0.75 (a 28% decline) over the 10-year average span between assessments (Reichborn-Kjennerud et al. 2015). This is a notable finding in part because both time points occurred in early adulthood, and the 10-year period does not cover critical developmental time periods that would be expected to demonstrate a change in personality. This finding is consistent with findings from clinical samples that demonstrated significant symptom reductions in patients who met categorical criteria over time, despite continuing to have some traits that might be viewed as pathological (Hopwood and Bleidorn 2018).

Second, ASPD is closely associated, although not synonymous, with criminal conduct. In practice, this means that once a person has been arrested for criminal conduct (whether convicted or not), which can be viewed as disregard for the rights of others, that qualifies the person for some of the criteria of ASPD for life because the past conduct does not change. However, decades of research demonstrate that criminal conduct does not continue at stable rates across the life span. Instead, almost all people desist from criminal conduct as they age. For instance, a nearly 70-year longitudinal follow-up study of 500 delinquent adolescent boys, first studied at an average age of 7 years, demonstrated that only 3% of those in the study continued to offend throughout adulthood, and even that small segment desisted by age 60 (Laub and Sampson 2009). Similarly, research that assessed 353 newly incarcerated men and women and then reassessed them 1 year later found that an ASPD diagnosis failed to predict future bad conduct in a custodial setting (Edens et al. 2015). Once an individual is labeled with ASPD, however, desistance from the behaviors is irrelevant to the continued diagnosis, which relies on historical conduct regardless of whether it continues or suggests future bad conduct. Thus, as the example of the adolescent exposed to lead at the beginning of this chapter suggests, once the acting-out behaviors become associated with a personality disorder label, that label will continue to stigmatize that individual in perpetuity, even when the cause of the behavior is a preventable toxic environmental exposure whose negative effects can be mitigated.

Third, findings from two longitudinal studies of people diagnosed with BPD indicate that most people with BPD recover, with the condition remitting for 85%–99% of subjects over 10–16 years of follow-up (Temes and Zanarini 2018). These two longitudinal studies recruited 465 patients with BPD and followed them prospectively. Patients with BPD were slower to remit than the comparison patients with major depression, but over time, the vast majority experienced extended periods of remission, with many being in remission for 8 or more years. Such findings have direct and important implications for how BPD is defined and diagnosed and raises substantive questions as to whether BPD is, in fact, enduring, pervasive, or inflexible as required by DSM-5's definition of a personality disorder. It is important to note that the majority of adults diagnosed with BPD are likely to have been physically or sexually abused or neglected as children and that childhood abuse increases the risk of an adulthood diagnosis of BPD four-fold (Johnson et al. 1999). Additionally, approximately 70% of individuals with BPD meet lifetime prevalence for major depressive disorder, and 88% meet lifetime prevalence for any anxiety disorder (Gunderson et al. 2018). This raises the question as to why the personality diagnoses supplant the psychiatric ones.

Finally, and perhaps most importantly for understanding the social inequity of personality disorder diagnoses, the DSM-5 field trials reported exceptionally poor interrater reliability and divergence for both ASPD and BPD. Interrater reliability is a measure of agreement between two (or more) independent evaluators when presented with the same evidence. High interrater reliability offers assurance that diagnostic categories and labels are not arbitrary and that they have meaning across assessment settings (such that different evaluators will arrive at the same diagnosis). The DSM-5 field trials found BPD to have a moderate level of agreement ($\kappa=0.54$) and ASPD to have a very poor level of agreement ($\kappa=0.21$) (Freedman et al. 2013). As discussed more below, these inadequate levels of agreement may result from bias, poor construct validity, or both, which raises doubts as to the scientific basis and meaning of ASPD and BPD.

Similarly, the failure to be able to distinguish personality disorders from each other, including ASPD and BPD, raises serious doubt as to what symptoms or behaviors are actually being assessed and whether the labels truly mean anything clinically. More than half of people who meet the criteria for any one personality disorder also meet the criteria for two or more personality disorders (Clark et al. 2018). This near-complete lack of specificity to the diagnoses suggests that the criteria are inadequate and/or the constructs lack validity. This lack of specificity increases the risk for bias in assessments because clinicians are left to their own feelings whether to assign one label versus another to a patient and raises doubt as to the validity of the constructs used to label people.

Moreover, ASPD and BPD may be diagnosed instead of (or co-occurring with) anxiety, depression, PTSD, mood disorders, and a host of other psychiatric illnesses. Some of these conditions may lead directly to behaviors that qualify a person for ASPD or BPD. They may also lead to self-medication and substance use disorders, which in turn lead to behaviors that qualify someone for ASPD or BPD. Research has shown that people of color are more likely to be perceived as behaviorally disordered than psychiatrically disordered (Mizock and Harkins 2011), which increases the likelihood of their being diagnosed with ASPD and BPD instead of the underlying psychiatric condition that is a cause of the behaviors.

Basically, problem behaviors observed in white children tend to be diagnosed as a psychiatric condition or simply accepted as youthful behavior, whereas the same problem behaviors in children of color often lead to a diagnosis of conduct disorder or oppositional defiant disorder, the predecessor conditions for ASPD. Similarly, girls and women are more likely to be characterized as having BPD when they either fail to conform or conform excessively to gender role stereotypes in therapeutic or clinical settings (i.e., appearing to a clinician to be overly dependent and needy, emotional, irrational, or manipulative). Women who manifest symptoms associated with being subjected to trauma, abuse, or assault are also more likely to be diagnosed with BPD because clinicians fail to view the long-term symptoms—such as difficulty trusting or conforming and adopting "correct" gender roles—in the historical context of traumatic experiences. This difference in how behaviors are perceived on the basis of the patient's race and gender contributes to unequal educational, social, medical, economic, and personal trajectories that may never be overcome.

A medical example may make this point more clearly. Hyperthyroidism is an easily diagnosable condition, detected by a simple blood test. However, the presentation of patients with hyperthyroidism often misdirects clinicians toward other issues. Hyperthyroidism is strongly associated with manic-like behavior, including nervousness, irritability, and impulsivity, as well as impaired decision making (Yuan et al. 2015). If the phenotype of the disease (i.e., the observable symptoms) is treated, the underlying thyroid disorder will remain untreated. This is the same conceptual problem as diagnosing or treating the phenotypes of ASPD and BPD as primary conditions or even co-occurring with psychiatric illnesses: it misses the underlying condition, the differential diagnoses, and the multiple possible causes of the observable symptoms.

Labeling and Stigma

If the consequence of being labeled with ASPD or BPD were beneficial or inconsequential, the poor reliability and validity would be largely a concern for psychometrists and statisticians. However, the consequences of being diagnosed with ASPD or BPD (or both)—labels that persist across the life span even when the symptoms do not—can be devastating. Labeling theory defines the ways in which stigma is created and maintained, reflecting a tendency to credit simple and immediate observations over structural and distal causes (Link and Phelan 1995). Thus, using the example at the beginning of the chapter, if a female adolescent receives a psychiatric evaluation because of disruptive, aggressive behaviors in class, the immediate observation would likely lead a clinician to consider that she has borderline personality traits, implying that the adolescent is impulsive, emotionally volatile, self-destructive, and overly sensitive to personal slights. Borderline personality traits as a label override and short-circuit the investigation of the developmental trajectory (which would uncover the lead exposure) and the social and structural underpinnings for why the adolescent was referred for an evaluation (which would uncover the increased risk for lead exposures on the basis of neighborhood factors, gender, race, and class).

This methodology is made most concrete in the approach of DSM-5 to the association between classist and coded racist language (e.g., low socioeconomic status, urban settings) and ASPD. As noted, DSM-5 acknowledges the association, but rather than identifying the root cause of the functional impairment as the problem, it opts for labeling the individual on the basis of the immediately observable behavior. In addition to the invalidity of the concept, this approach takes identified and known structural causes of functional impairments and, rather than addressing those causes, blames the very people who have been disadvantaged by those structural inequities (Hardeman et al. 2016). This is worsened by the evidence that the label itself causes stigma, meaning that even when the behaviors no longer exist or are statistically controlled in research studies, the label is enough without the behavior to increase stigma (Pescosolido 2013), thereby reinforcing the very inequity that caused the impairment in the first place.

The consequences of an inaccurate label may also be severe. For instance, a woman who was sexually assaulted as an adolescent may, as an adult, develop symptoms that could be construed as BPD: self-harm, difficulty entering into trusting relationships, depression, anxiety, and/or hostility. Clinicians may be reluctant to treat patients they view as having BPD (Bodner et al. 2015), believing them to be treatment resistant, manipulative, and extremely challenging to manage. Thus, the BPD label in a medical chart increases the chance of worse access to health care because clinicians may seek to avoid people so labeled, a situation that likely deters people with functional impairments from seeking care and increases the likelihood of inaccurate assessments. Moreover, this hypothetical woman may be suffering from the long-term consequences of trauma, and she can be effectively treated. The difference between being labeled with a treatable mental illness (a condition that a person has) and a personality disorder (a character flaw that defines a person) is consequential in every way for the patient.

Assessment of Personality Disorders

How ASPD and BPD are assessed or measured raises further questions about what the diagnoses mean and the consequences they have on patients. Two approaches predominate: the clinical interview and the use of personality tests. The assessments that lead to consideration of personality disorders are limited and generally nonscientific.

The Clinical Interview

The standard approach typically relies on a personal interview and assessing the patient's self-report. That self-report may or may not include answering questions on a structured test. The current practice involves talking to a patient, with little attention given either to recognizing and avoiding one's own biases or to collecting and interpreting all available collateral evidence. For a host of reasons, a patient may not be a good reporter of his or her own experiences, may be reluctant to disclose some information, may be unaware of what is relevant or important, or may have limited insight into the symptoms experienced. Lack of trust and rapport, in addition to the context of the evaluation (which may occur for reasons other than the individual's seeking support or treatment), should caution clinicians against giving too much weight to the *facts* elicited during the interview and should guide them toward establishing a common understanding, language, and therapeutic alliance (Ramsden 2018). For instance, without having established a substantial level of rapport and trust, a patient with BPD may be especially unwilling to disclose the abuse history that could be a major contributing factor to the symptoms experienced.

Additionally, clinician biases may render the clinical interview suspect. This bias can be both explicit and implicit, and it is worsened in the case of an ahistorical, noncontextual assessment (Iudici et al. 2015), even when clinicians believe they are bias-free (Neal and Brodsky 2016). In a review of bias in psychological evaluations, Neal and Grisso (2014) reported on the scope and potential effect of examiner bias and defined it as a type of systematic (rather than random) error. The idea of bias as a systematic error helps frame its effects on assessment. There are three common forms of systematic unreliability: cultural overshadowing, expectation bias, and confirmation bias. *Cultural overshadowing* occurs when a clinician does not see or denies the true biological or psychological condition of the individual being assessed because of specific sociocultural characteristics (e.g., poverty, race, gender, immigration status) (Friedman 2017; Woods et al. 2011). In other words, the clinician's expectations, often based on stereotyped information about a group to which the patient belongs, short-circuits the process of gathering reliable and valid information. For instance, the belief that Black people experience less pain than white people, a stereotyped belief that originated as a justification for the enslavement of Black people, overshadows the necessary clinical determination of the level of pain a specific patient experiences and the correct treatment needed (Hoffman et al. 2016). For Black men, this stereotype leads to assumptions about criminality and ASPD; for Black women, it leads to denial of care and assumptions about attention-seeking and BPD.

Expectation bias may derive from political or social beliefs, such as the belief that people who are arrested are guilty of something, even if not the specific crime for which they were arrested, or from the belief that people of certain racial or economic statuses are more likely to commit crimes. This may be an explicit or implicit belief. In this way, a clinician's implicit or explicit racial bias that men of color are dangerous is reformulated as the patient's personality disorder, more likely culminating in a pejorative label and recasting of the patient's behavior in light of the belief that the person is dangerous. For example, one aspect of the diagnostic criterion "[f]ailure to conform to social norms" can be truancy from school. A clinician might ask whether the patient regularly missed school, and if the answer is yes, might consider that as evidence supporting a disregard for social norms and rules. A clinician performing an unbiased evaluation would also seek to understand *why* the patient missed school: Was the patient unable to get to school? Ashamed because they were cognitively impaired and unable to keep up with their classmates? Had to work to support their family? Such information might recast the disregard for norms as a commitment to financially supporting one's family despite the risk of being truant or a reflection of the need for academic supports.

Confirmation bias occurs, for example, when a clinician expects that a person with a history of carceral system involvement or a person of a certain sociodemographic background is going to meet criteria for ASPD and then seeks out confirmation, ignoring or not seeking data that do not support that hypothesis (Freedman and Zaami 2019). In the case of personality disorders, confirmation bias regarding gender may lead a clinician to assume that women have BPD and men have ASPD, reflecting the cultural bias that women internalize and men externalize, and then to pursue anecdotal, decontextualized behaviors to prove the point while ignoring the complexity of how context shapes behavior. Confirmation bias also influences the use and selection of symptom rating scales. On the one hand, if a clinician has no suspicion whatsoever that a white female patient with mood and psychotic symptoms has schizophrenia, the clinician is less likely to use the schizophrenia scale during the assessment. On the other hand, if a clinician suspects that a Black male patient with mood and psychotic symptoms has schizophrenia, the clinician is more likely to use the schizophrenia scale during the assessment.

Personality Test Instruments

In addition to clinical interviewing to assess personality, self-report test instruments are commonly used. Many hundreds of these instruments exist and are for sale, but a handful are more commonly used, most often one of the versions of the Minnesota Multiphasic Personality Inventory–2 (MMPI-2; Butcher et al. 2001) or the Personality Assessment Inventory–2 (PAI-2; Morey 2007). The scales of these instruments are intended to reflect traits, not symptoms, meaning those characteristics that are usually said to be impervious to change or intervention. Some of the measures include scales that sound diagnostic (e.g., both the MMPI-2 and PAI-2 have Schizophrenia scales), but the test manuals carefully advise that an elevated clinical scale score is insufficient to diagnose a person and may only be tangentially related to the symptoms that are required for diagnosis. Thus, an elevated Schizophrenia scale score does not mean the person has schizophrenia, and an elevated Antisocial scale score does not mean the person meets criteria for ASPD.

The vast literature using these instruments can make it difficult to understand the research on their psychometric reliability and validity. Debate regarding cultural biases of the questions and differential answering by race continues, but both the PAI-2 and MMPI-2 show differences by race on questions related to infrequently endorsed symptoms (i.e., questions to which most people give the same answer but the current respondent answers in an unusual manner), as well as anxiety, schizophrenia, paranoia, stress, warmth, antisociality, mania, bizarre mentation, and anger (Arbisi et al. 2002; Estrada and Smith 2019; Hill et al. 2012). In a direct comparison of 1,411 Black and white veterans in treatment for substance use, Black veterans' scores on some key MMPI-2 scales, including antisocial, fears, cynicism, and bizarre mentation, were significantly higher. This finding clearly suggests racial bias problems with the test instrument (Monnot et al. 2009). Gender bias has also been reported on the MMPI-2–Restructured Form, with higher percentages of women found to be malingering because on average they endorse uncommon virtues (i.e., they present themselves in an overly positive way compared with expectation) and minimize pathological symptoms (Mazza et al. 2019). Notably, social desirability, as potentially reflected by endorsing uncommon virtue and underreporting pathology, is a gendered expectation and should be evaluated as a patriarchal cultural pressure and expectation of women, rather than an attempt by women to deceive or "fake good."

Equally as significant, the test-retest reliability of these instruments suggests that either they are poor measures of many of the conditions they purport to assess or the conditions are temporary and subject to large changes in a short period of time. Test-retest reliability compares the same subject taking the same test at two different time points. Differences in the results at the two time points suggest either measurement error or changes in the underlying condition. With the MMPI-2, only 28% of scales performed adequately on this basic measure of reliability, which means that many of the clinical scales, restructured scales, personality scales, and content scales have low reliability, some so low as to raise doubt as to whether they have any merit whatsoever or should be interpreted at all (Wise et al. 2010). Low reliability poses the biggest problem for the interpretation of the clinical scales. Test-retest reliability on the PAI-2 is reported to be better but also varies by scale, ranging between 0.68 and 0.92, with a number of the malingering and effort scales having lower reliability (Strauss et al. 2006).

It is surprising that ASPD test-retest reliability would not be very high because many of the criteria for its diagnosis are static—*once met, always met*. Overall, however, the instruments most often used to determine whether a person has a personality disorder are seriously flawed when it comes to understanding and interpreting the significance of the results, which appear to be at best a snapshot of current functioning rather than a description of an inflexible and stable personality disorder as required by the diagnostic criteria.

Although these assessment instruments are used widely for a variety of purposes, in clinical and forensic settings, typically they are used to discount serious mental illnesses, dehumanize and create distance, imply a predisposition to future problematic behavior because of a character flaw, and suggest that the person cannot benefit from treatment (Wayland and O'Brien 2013). They often are used without an understanding of their psychometric limitations or the influence of race, class, and gender bias in their design. The language of personality disorders that these tests justify using is that the person is characterologically flawed and irredeemable, rather than that the person has an illness and acted in a specific context. These tests, then, help to reframe the structural inequity of race, class, gender, and discrimination as an individual's failures to adapt and conform.

The Individualistic Fallacy

One of the central problems with assessments of personality disorders is that they "locate" the problem within the individual, disregarding the structural, environmental, and distal forces at play. For instance, diagnoses of personality disorders as a way to explain behavior suggest that the problem is how a person responds to the experience of racism, not the racism itself. This is sometimes referred to as the *individualistic fallacy*, which assumes that individual-level outcomes (behavior, functioning) should be attributed solely to individual characteristics or traits (personality), thereby fundamentally denying the structural, social, institutional, contextual, and environmental frame within which behaviors and functioning occur (Silver 2000). Said another way, the individualistic fallacy assigns a causal role to only those elements that are proximate and are immediately observable, when in fact the causes of behavior and functioning are complex, accumulate and vary across the developmental and life span trajectory, and are shaped in historical, political, social, and environmental contexts.

This approach identifies the individual as their own cause for impaired or disordered functioning (i.e., flawed character) and serves as a means of social control that maintains the status quo by actively ignoring distal and structural causes (e.g., racism, sexism, poverty, discrimination) as they come to bear in context. DSM-5 contributes to this process by describing a higher prevalence of ASPD among those affected by poverty and sociocultural factors, while maintaining that the disorder is an *inner experience*, thereby explicitly setting out that the problem is *only* the person and not the poverty, racism, sexism, and discrimination. DSM-5 fails to consider how or why poverty or sociocultural factors contribute and then ignores them entirely in the discussion about diagnosis, which is focused on the individual's failures as a person. This approach explicitly dehumanizes the person subjected to structural oppression, worsening the stigma and maintaining structural inequity. Furthermore, it ignores the extensive scientific literature on the causal relationship between poverty, discrimination, trauma, and psychiatric illnesses (Bogart et al. 2013; Gur et al. 2019; Sibrava et al. 2019).

This approach is especially problematic for ASPD, which draws on interactions with the carceral system as part of the framework that may qualify a person for the disorder. According to a criminology theory that dates to the early 1990s, a demographic boom was creating an inevitable cohort of Black juvenile "super-predators" who would terrorize American cities (Dilulio 2005). This theory, widely endorsed at the time but since renounced by its primary architects, was critical in offering what was purported to be *scientific* support for the implementation of public policy that explicitly worsened the mass incarceration crisis (Alexander 2012), and the theory drew explicitly on racist stereotypes and white fear, which originated in the justifications for slavery and colonialism (Atkins-Loria et al. 2015).

The criminalization of Black youth as a group increases the likelihood that individual young Black men will be diagnosed with ASPD because they are drawn disproportionately into the carceral system by policy. Thus, stop-and-frisk policing—the practice of physically detaining and searching people on the street who have not engaged in criminal or suspect behaviors but who police believe to be potentially more likely to do so at some future time—leads to increased contacts and increased arrests of young men of color, which leads to a greater risk of a law enforcement record, which then suggests a "failure to conform to social norms with respect to lawful behaviors, as indicated by repeatedly performing acts that are grounds for arrest" (American Psychiatric Association 2013, p. 659). As more children, women, and men of color and poor people are drawn into the carceral system in response to policy changes, their chance of being labeled as having ASPD increases, thereby also increasing the likelihood of a longer duration within the carceral system. In actuality, the stop-and-frisk policy is strongly associated with increased trauma and anxiety among the young men of color most subjected to it (Geller et al. 2014).

Because of this social policy, a diagnosis such as ASPD, which relies on criminal history, will by definition be inequitable on the basis of race and class. People of color and poor people have disproportionate numbers of police contacts, detentions, and arrests; longer and harsher sentences; and worse access to medical and psychiatric care in custodial settings. Because the ASPD diagnosis takes precedence, it leads to a greater likelihood of custodial infractions; greater barriers to community reentry and to obtaining housing, employment, services, and support; and a greater risk of re-arrest (Del Toro et al. 2019; Lamb and Weinberger 2013; Liberman et al. 2014; Weaver and Geller 2019). Once a person is labeled as having ASPD, this process is worsened because, despite the evidence discussed above that ASPD is not a reliable or valid predictor of future conduct, carceral institutions rely on the diagnosis.

From Social Context to the Individual

The process by which social institutions—and the mental health professionals working within these institutions—regard structural causes of inequity as the fault of the individual sustains structural inequity. Said another way, it is a key mechanism by which structural inequity maintains itself. If the individual who "fails" to adjust to being discriminated against is at fault for not adjusting, rather than the problem being one of inequity and discrimination, the individual can be labeled, stigmatized, and defined as less than human, leaving in place the structural barriers to equity. Character and personality are at fault for not adjusting adequately to being oppressed. Quite simply, if the problem is character, there is little to do but blame the individual. If the problem is structural, the solution is complicated and requires social and structural changes, as well as a therapeutic alliance with the patient that recognizes the historical and current context of the psychological trauma the individual experiences. A predominant function, whether intended or not, of personality disorders such as ASPD and BPD, appears to be the maintenance and replication of structural inequities that seek to label and stigmatize through psychiatric diagnoses.

When is it Appropriate to Diagnose a Personality Disorder?

Given the foregoing discussion, any clinical diagnosis or assessment of personality disorders should be approached cautiously. First and foremost, personality disorders should not be diagnosed when a patient has a psychiatric, neurological, or medical condition. As discussed, personality disorders are not merely add-ons or co-occurring disorders. The lack of reliability and validity, the influence of bias in the assessment, and the significant risk of failing to identify treatable psychiatric, neurological, and medical conditions all lead toward not including ASPD and BPD in the diagnostic framework. This does not mean that the clinician will not feel or believe that a patient's personality is a barrier, but it is recommended that the clinician's feelings or beliefs be put aside in the formal assessment process because of the noted failures of the conceptualization and the significant limits of its assessment. If trauma is the cause of a patient's symptoms that appear to be BPD or ASPD, the clinician should diagnose and treat the trauma. If problematic behaviors interfere with a patient's ability to function, the clinician should identify and address those behaviors with therapeutic interventions such as dialectical behavior therapy or multisystemic therapy.

Second, mental health professionals must make themselves aware: aware of the limits of the personality construct; aware of their own biases, both implicit and explicit; and aware of the role of personality diagnoses in maintaining social inequity and increasing stigma. Toward this goal, clinicians need to participate in an ongoing continuing education process through which they increase their structural competence to make themselves aware of the historical context of each patient, as well as more generally learn how structural inequity works and interferes with a patient's functioning (Metzl and Hansen 2014). Especially in high-stakes assessment settings, this is one key component to a best-practices approach.

Finally, in working toward improving structural competence, mental health professionals will become better equipped at documenting and explaining structural inequity. This should become a core part of the education of new practitioners, as well as a core component of assessment, treatment, and documentation. Recognizing the mechanisms by which structural and distal causes affect the daily behavior and functioning of patients is also a best-practices approach. Mental health professionals need to recognize the individualistic fallacy and make substantial effort to avoid it. Psychiatrists can make a substantial contribution toward improving structural humility, and they can work to change the structural inequities underlying, and reinforced by, the diagnoses of ASPD and BPD.

Questions for Self-Reflection

1. What are my associations (implicit and explicit) about people with antisocial personality disorder? About people with borderline personality disorder?
2. Are there patterns in my diagnosis (or suspicion of diagnosis) of people with antisocial and borderline personality disorders by race? By gender? To what do I attribute these patterns?
3. How do I feel about the authors' assertion that personality disorder diagnoses can harm patients?

References

Alexander M: The New Jim Crow: Mass Incarceration in the Age of Colorblindness. New York, New Press, 2012

American Psychiatric Association: Diagnostic and Statistical Manual of Mental Disorders, 5th Edition. Arlington, VA, American Psychiatric Association, 2013

Arbisi PA, Ben-Porath YS, McNulty J: A comparison of MMPI-2 validity in African American and Caucasian psychiatric inpatients. Psychol Assess 14:3–15, 2002

Atkins-Loria S, Macdonald H, Mitterling C: Young African American men and the diagnosis of conduct disorder: the neo-colonization of suffering. Clin Soc Work J 43:431–441, 2015

Bodner E, Cohen-Fridel S, Mashiah M, et al: The attitudes of psychiatric hospital staff toward hospitalization and treatment of patients with borderline personality disorder. BMC Psychiatry 15:2, 2015

Bogart LM, Elliott MN, Kanouse DE, et al: Association between perceived discrimination and racial/ethnic disparities in problem behaviors among preadolescent youths. Am J Public Health 103:1074–1081, 2013

Butcher JN, Graham JR, Ben-Porath YS, et al: MMPI-2 (Minnesota Multiphasic Personality Inventory 2): Manual for Administration, Scoring, and Interpretation, Revised Edition. Minneapolis, MN, University of Minnesota Press, 2001

Clark LA, Nuzum H, Ro E: Manifestations of personality impairment severity: comorbidity, course/prognosis, psychosocial dysfunction, and "borderline" personality features. Curr Opin Psychol 21:117–121, 2018

Del Toro J, Lloyd T, Buchanan KS, et al: The criminogenic and psychological effects of police stops on adolescent black and Latino boys. Proc Natl Acad Sci 116:8261–8268, 2019

Dilulio J: My black crime problem, and ours, in Race, Crime, and Justice: A Reader. Edited by Gabbidon SL, Greene HT. New York, Routledge, 2005, pp 73–96

Edens JF, Kelley SE, Lilienfeld SO, et al: DSM-5 antisocial personality disorder: predictive validity in a prison sample. Law Hum Behav 39:123–129, 2015

Estrada AR, Smith SR: An exploration of Latina/o respondent scores on the Personality Assessment Inventory. Curr Psychol 38:782–791, 2019

Freedman D, Zaami S: Neuroscience and mental state issues in forensic assessment. Int J Law Psychiatry 65:101437, 2019

Freedman R, Lewis DA, Michels R, et al: The initial field trials of DSM-5: new blooms and old thorns. Am J Psychiatry 170:1–5, 2013

Friedman SH: Culture, bias, and understanding: we can do better. J Am Acad Psychiatry Law 45:136–139, 2017

Geller A, Fagan J, Tyler T, Link BG: Aggressive policing and the mental health of young urban men. Am J Public Health 104:2321–2327, 2014

Gunderson JG, Herpertz SC, Skodol AE, et al: Borderline personality disorder. Nat Rev Dis Primers 4:18029, 2018

Gur RE, Moore TM, Rosen AFG, et al: Burden of environmental adversity associated with psychopathology, maturation, and brain behavior parameters in youths. JAMA Psychiatry 76:966–975, 2019

Hardeman RR, Medina EM, Kozhimannil KB: Structural racism and supporting black lives—the role of health professionals. N Engl J Med 375:2113–2115, 2016

Hill JS, Robbins RR, Pace TM: Cultural validity of the Minnesota Multiphasic Personality Inventory–2 empirical correlates: is this the best we can do? J Multicult Couns Devel 40:104–116, 2012

Hoffman KM, Trawalter S, Axt JR, Oliver MN: Racial bias in pain assessment and treatment recommendations, and false beliefs about biological differences between blacks and whites. Proc Natl Acad Sci 113:4296–4301, 2016

Hopwood CJ, Bleidorn W: Stability and change in personality and personality disorders. Curr Opin Psychol 21:6–10, 2018

Iudici A, Salvini A, Faccio E, Castelnuovo G: The clinical assessment in the legal field: an empirical study of bias and limitations in forensic expertise. Front Psychol 6:1831, 2015

Johnson JG, Cohen P, Brown J, et al: Childhood maltreatment increases risk for personality disorders during early adulthood. Arch Gen Psychiatry 56:600–606, 1999

Lamb HR, Weinberger LE: Some perspectives on criminalization. J Am Acad Psychiatry Law 41:287–293, 2013

Laub JH, Sampson RJ: Shared Beginnings, Divergent Lives. Boston, MA, Harvard University Press, 2009

Liberman AM, Kirk DS, Kim K: Labeling effects of first juvenile arrests: secondary deviance and secondary sanctioning. Criminology 52:345–370, 2014

Link BG, Phelan J: Social conditions as fundamental causes of disease. J Health Soc Behav (spec):80–94, 1995

Mazza C, Burla F, Verrocchio MC, et al: MMPI-2-RF profiles in child custody litigants. Front Psychiatry 10:725, 2019

Metzl JM, Hansen H: Structural competency: theorizing a new medical engagement with stigma and inequality. Soc Sci Med.103:126–133, 2014

Mizock L, Harkins D: Diagnostic bias and conduct disorder: improving culturally sensitive diagnosis. Child Youth Serv 32:243–253, 2011

Monnot MJ, Quirk SW, Hoerger M, Brewer L: Racial bias in personality assessment: using the MMPI-2 to predict psychiatric diagnoses of African American and Caucasian chemical dependency inpatients. Psychol Assess 21:137–151, 2009

Morey LC: Personality Assessment Inventory Professional Manual, 2nd Edition. Lutz, FL, Psychological Assessment Resources, 2007

Neal TMS, Brodsky SL: Forensic psychologists' perceptions of bias and potential correction strategies in forensic mental health evaluations. Psychol Public Policy Law 22:58–76, 2016

Neal TMS, Grisso T: The cognitive underpinnings of bias in forensic mental health evaluations. Psychol Public Policy Law 20:200–211, 2014

Pescosolido BA: The public stigma of mental illness: what do we think; what do we know; what can we prove? J Health Soc Behav 54:1–21, 2013

Ramsden J: "Are you calling me a liar"? Clinical interviewing more for trust than knowledge with high-risk men with antisocial personality disorder. Int J Forensic Ment Health 17:351–361, 2018

Reichborn-Kjennerud T, Czajkowski N, Ystrom E, et al: A longitudinal twin study of borderline and antisocial personality disorder traits in early to middle adulthood. Psychol Med 45:3121–3131, 2015

Sibrava NJ, Bjornsson AS, Perez Benitez ACI, et al: Posttraumatic stress disorder in African American and Latinx adults: clinical course and the role of racial and ethnic discrimination. Am Psychol 74:101–116, 2019

Silver E: Race, neighborhood disadvantage, and violence among persons with mental disorders: the importance of contextual measurement. Law Hum Behav 24:449–456, 2000

Strauss EE, Sherman EMS, Spreen O: A Compendium of Neuropsychological Tests: Administration, Norms, and Commentary. New York, Oxford University Press, 2006

Temes CM, Zanarini MC: The longitudinal course of borderline personality disorder. Psychiatr Clin North Am 41:685–694, 2018

Wayland K, O'Brien SD: Deconstructing antisocial personality disorder and psychopathy: a guidelines-based approach to prejudicial psychiatric labels. Hofstra Law Rev 42:519–588, 2013

Weaver VM, Geller A: De-policing America's youth: disrupting criminal justice policy feedbacks that distort power and derail prospects. Ann Am Acad Pol Soc Sci 685:190–226, 2019

Wise EA, Streiner DL, Walfish S: A review and comparison of the reliabilities of the MMPI-2, MCMI-III, and PAI presented in their respective test manuals. Meas Eval Couns Dev 42:246–254, 2010

Woods GW, Greenspan S, Agharkar BS: Ethnic and cultural factors in identifying fetal alcohol spectrum disorders. J Psychiatry Law 39:9–37, 2011

Yuan L, Tian Y, Zhang F, et al: Decision-making in patients with hyperthyroidism: a neuropsychological study. PLoS One 10(6):e0129773, 2015

CHAPTER 13

Social Injustice and Child Trauma

Walter E. Wilson Jr., M.D., M.H.A.
Nicole Cotton, M.D.
Sarah Y. Vinson, M.D.

> The developing child's positive sense of self depends on the caregiver's benign use of power.
>
> *Judith Herman*

Trauma research tells what *should* be a compelling story: childhood trauma can distort psychological development, precipitate child and adult psychopathology, and skew life trajectories. Yet, in an American society equipped with both this knowledge and vast resources that could be employed to limit trauma's reach, trauma is permitted to play a prominent role in the lives of many children, adolescents, and families. A thorough exploration of this phenomenon requires the acknowledgment of trauma's various forms. Particularly for clinicians, a critical appraisal of traditional psychiatric conceptualizations of trauma's many manifestations is also indicated. Childhood trauma caused by experiences in the home (e.g., physical abuse, sexual abuse, exposure to domestic violence) or by isolated events (e.g., natural disasters, motor vehicle accidents) are frequently areas of focus for both clinicians and the larger society. This approach, however, overlooks what is often the most pervasive, unrelenting, and pernicious form of trauma affecting marginalized populations: structural trauma.

Interpersonal traumas can be attributed to individual bad actors. Accidents are the result of exceptions or malfunctions. With structural trauma, however, society's systems as they are intentionally configured and regularly operate are the instruments of harm. The social determinants of mental health and the systemic structures that frame them are powerful forces in the psychological development and well-being of children, a vulnerable population that is, by definition, legally dependent on either a family or the child welfare system to meet its basic needs. When it comes to the consideration of these structural issues, both the typical child trauma assessment techniques and psychiatric diagnoses have critical omissions. Just as childhood dysfunction cannot be understood apart from the context of family violence and neglect, family dysfunction cannot be understood apart from the context of societal violence and neglect.

The Adverse Childhood Experiences Studies

One of the most referenced and well-known studies regarding childhood trauma is the Adverse Childhood Experiences Study (ACE Study), originally conducted beginning in 1995. It explored the relationship between childhood abuse and household dysfunction and later-life medical conditions that lead to premature death in adults. The initial study included information from 9,508 respondents, 80% of whom were white and 75% of whom had at least some college education. Participants completed the Adverse Childhood Experience Questionnaire (Table 13–1). Results indicated that adverse childhood experiences (ACEs) were common in this largely middle-class population (Felitti et al. 1998). Although the finding that childhood trauma increases the risk of mental illness was not novel, the ACE Study's demonstration of a dose-response relationship between childhood trauma and a wide range of outcomes in adult physical health, mental health, and psychosocial functioning cemented its status as a landmark study (Centers for Disease Control and Prevention 2020). Key findings of that ACE Study are provided in Figure 13–1.

Following the original ACE Study, a larger study of 214,157 people with greater socioeconomic and racial diversity was conducted in 2011–2014, using a slightly modified version of the ACE questionnaire and data

TABLE 13–1. Original Adverse Childhood Experiences (ACE) Questionnaire

While you were growing up, during your first 18 years of life:

1. Did a parent or other adult in the household **often**...

   Swear at you, insult you, put you down, or humiliate you?

   or

   Act in a way that made you afraid that you might be physically hurt?

   Yes   No   If yes enter 1 ____

2. Did a parent or other adult in the household **often**...

   Push, grab, slap, or throw something at you?

   or

   Ever hit you so hard that you had marks or were injured?

   Yes   No   If yes enter 1 ____

3. Did an adult or person at least 5 years older than you **ever**...

   Touch or fondle you or have you touch their body in a sexual way?

   or

   Try to or actually have oral, anal, or vaginal sex with you?

   Yes   No   If yes enter 1 ____

4. Did you **often** feel that...

   No one in your family loved you or thought you were important or special?

   or

   Your family didn't look out for each other, feel close to each other, or support each other?

   Yes   No   If yes enter 1 ____

5. Did you **often** feel that...

   You didn't have enough to eat, had to wear dirty clothes, and had no one to protect you?

   or

   Your parents were too drunk or high to take care of you or take you to the doctor if you needed it?

   Yes   No   If yes enter 1 ____

TABLE 13–1. Original Adverse Childhood Experiences (ACE) Questionnaire *(continued)*

6. Were your parents **ever** separated or divorced?

   Yes   No   If yes enter 1 ___

7. Was your mother or stepmother:

   Often pushed, grabbed, slapped, or had something thrown at her?

   or

   Sometimes or often kicked, bitten, hit with a fist, or hit with something hard?

   or

   Ever repeatedly hit over at least a few minutes or threatened with a gun or knife?

   Yes   No   If yes enter 1 ___

8. Did you live with anyone who was a problem drinker or alcoholic or who used street drugs?

   Yes   No   If yes enter 1 ___

9. Was a household member depressed or mentally ill or did a household member attempt suicide?

   Yes   No   If yes enter 1 ___

10. Did a household member go to prison?

   Yes   No   If yes enter 1 ___

Now add up your "Yes" answers: _____. This is your ACE score.

Note. The ACE Study looked at three categories of adverse experience: *childhood abuse,* which included emotional, physical, and sexual abuse; *neglect,* including both physical and emotional neglect; and *household challenges,* which included growing up in a household where there was substance abuse, mental illness, violent treatment of a mother or stepmother, or parental separation/divorce or a member of the household went to prison. Respondents were given an ACE score between 0 and 10 on the basis of how many of these 10 types of adverse experiences to which they reported being exposed.

from the Behavioral Risk Factor Surveillance System (BRFSS). Modification included making abuse questions more appropriate for a telephone survey and broadening the question related to intimate partner violence to include any parent or adult. The results reflected an even higher prevalence of childhood abuse and markers of family dysfunction than in the original study. Additionally, traumatic exposures were substantially higher for Black, Latinx, and multiracial respondents, as well as for those with less than a high school education and with less than $15,000 annual family in-

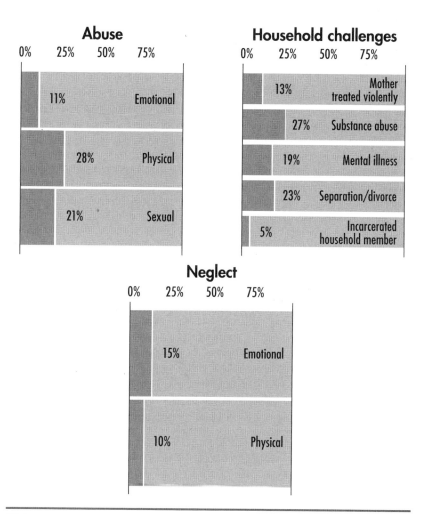

FIGURE 13–1. Adverse Childhood Experiences Study (ACE Study) by Merrick et al. 2018: general findings.

Source. Reproduced from Centers for Disease Control and Prevention, Kaiser Permanente: *The ACE Study Survey Data.* Atlanta, GA, U.S. Department of Health and Human Services, Centers for Disease Control and Prevention, 2016.

come. Figure 13–2 provides key findings of this modified ACE Study. Of note, approximately 25% of individuals surveyed reported three or more ACEs. This study highlights that although common across groups, the burden of childhood adversity is distributed inequitably (Merrick et al. 2018).

Although the ACE Study and BRFSS study have achieved a place of preeminence in the professional and lay discourse regarding trauma, the approach used in these studies does not take into account community vio-

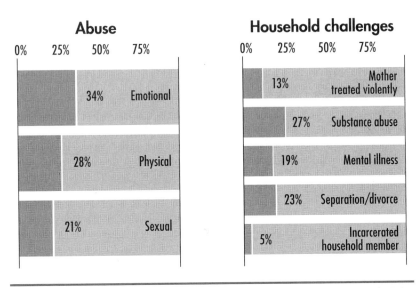

FIGURE 13–2.   ACE module from the 2011–2014 Behavioral Risk Factor Surveillance System (BRFSS): key findings.

Source.   Merrick MT, Ford DC, Ports KA, Guinn AS: "Prevalence of adverse childhood experiences from the 2011–2014 Behavioral Risk Factor Surveillance System in 23 States." *JAMA Pediatrics* 172(11):1036–1044, 2018.

lence, structural trauma, racial trauma, or the severity and chronicity of trauma. The questionnaire captures individual issues that impair the caregiver (e.g., whether the parent has an alcohol use disorder or mental illness that could hinder proper child care [Felitti et al. 1998]), but it gives no consideration to societal drivers of parental dysfunction (e.g., whether the caregiver's drinking is a method to cope with distress related to his or her own trauma or whether the caregiver has an untreated mental illness because the safety net clinic has a 3-month waitlist). Furthermore, the original questionnaire presumes a family structure in which the mother or stepmother is the primary caregiver. Although these omissions may not have been particularly relevant for the original study's largely white, middle-class study population, they certainly would be for Black, brown, and impoverished children who have faced familial disruption in the context of structural racism and traumatized communities.

Researchers have since looked beyond conventional ACEs, in attempts to understand expanded ACEs affecting socioeconomically and racially diverse populations. These *expanded ACEs* include, for example, witnessing violence, experiencing discrimination, growing up in unsafe neighborhoods, experiencing bullying, and living in foster care (Cronholm et al.

2015). Importantly, although there has been some expansion of the questions used in ACE surveys to more accurately reflect the experiences of marginalized populations (Chen and Burke Harris 2014), in clinical practice and lay discussion, the original 10-question survey of conventional ACEs is the one most widely used.

Community Violence

Community violence includes extreme events such as shootings, stabbings, and sexual assault but also can include less severe, more pervasive events such as drug deals and robberies. Exposure to community violence can be direct (e.g., the child is attacked) or indirect (e.g., the child witnesses a shooting). In communities where violence is routine, both children and the adults entrusted with their care (who may themselves have been exposed as children) are continuously subjected to threats against their well-being. High-quality parenting practices and the reestablishment of a sense of safety are important strategies for protecting children from traumatic exposures and bolstering resilience following adverse events. It can be challenging for parents to provide a sense of safety for their children when the parents also are not safe; therefore, it is hardly surprising that parental trauma, distress, and PTSD diagnoses correlate with an increased risk of children experiencing child abuse or being diagnosed with PTSD (Cross et al. 2018). When rapid brain growth and increased neuroplasticity occur in youth in this context of toxic stress, it follows that such environments can have a direct, negative psychobiological impact on the developing neurological systems of children and adolescents (DeBellis 2001).

Many children in the United States experience community violence; however, urban and poor youth are disproportionately affected. Additionally, young people of color who are already contending with inequities and stressors from structural and interpersonal racism are more likely to live in these environments. Even ACE questionnaires that do not directly ask about these issues capture the disproportionate impact of trauma experienced by minority urban youth; research suggests that Black adolescents are victims of trauma at a rate that is 67% higher than for white adolescents (Sabol et al. 2004). In one study of racially diverse, poor mothers and their children in Massachusetts, more than 30% of children reported having witnessed violence at school or in their neighborhood, 38% reported worrying about a robbery or burglary of their home or family, and 30% reported worrying about their safety where they live (Mohammad et al. 2015). In a study of young Black men ages 18–24 in Baltimore, Maryland, participants reported knowing an average of three homicide victims, the majority of whom were peers (Smith 2015). Findings from the National Crime Victimization Survey show that the risk of experiencing serious violence is roughly 1.5–2 times greater for Blacks than for whites, and the risk for Latinx people is roughly 1.2–1.5 times greater than for whites (Warnken and Lauritsen 2019). These experiences have psychiatric manifestations, including behavioral and emotional dysregulation, PTSD symptoms, depression, and suicidality, as well as social manifestations, including poor academic performance, higher rates of homelessness, and increased risk for criminal justice system involvement (Carrion et al. 2002; Edalati et al. 2017; Felitti et al. 1998; Roos et al. 2013).

Poverty as a Mediator for Child Social Determinants of Health

Per developmental systems theory, healthy and successful child development is more likely when children can access environmental resources in communities rich in assets aligned with their individual strengths (Benson 2003). This is not the reality for children living in poverty, who make up a significant portion of the U.S. population. Approximately 21% of all children (a number that corresponds to roughly 15 million developing brains) are members of households living below the federal poverty line—a benchmark set at an annual income of $26,200 for a family of four in 2020 (Office of the Assistant Secretary for Planning and Evaluation 2020). Another 43% of U.S. children live in low-income families, defined as having incomes less than twice the federal poverty line (National Center for Children in Poverty 2019). Although more white children live in poverty than any other group, higher proportions of Black, Hispanic, and American Indian/Alaska Native children do; 34% of Black children, 28% of Hispanic children, and 34% of American Indian/Alaska Native children live in poverty, compared with 11% of both white and Asian children (National Center for Education Statistics 2017). However, because these data represent averages across subgroups with substantial heterogeneity, they are misleading for certain subgroups. For example, one in three Hmong children in the United States live in poverty (Asian American Federation 2014), a rate far higher than the broader Asian racial group in which they are categorized.

As highlighted throughout this chapter, social determinants of mental health have clear clinical implications for traumatized youth, and poverty is a frequent and powerful mediator of social determinants. The World Health Organization (Solar and Irwin 2010) identified several key concepts from Finn Diderichsen's model of the mechanisms of health inequality that help explain the relationship between social status and health outcomes:

- Social contexts create social stratification and assign individuals to different social positions
- Social stratification, in turn, engenders a differential exposure to health-damaging conditions and differential vulnerability in terms of health conditions and material resource availability
- Social stratification determines differential consequences of ill health for more and less advantaged groups

This theoretical framework is helpful for understanding and addressing childhood trauma in a society shaped by structural oppression, be it based on gender, race, economic status, or other demographic categories.

The following case introduces a mother and son who both experienced childhood structural trauma. We refer back to this family in the remainder of this section.

Case Example

David, a 4-year-old multiracial boy, is called "defiant" in school because he does not follow teachers' instructions. He reacts impulsively when upset and has hit other children on several occasions. He is referred by his pre-school for a mental health evaluation. His mother, Ava, describes him as a bright, energetic, loving son. In the office, he is noted to be pleasant and engaging. On approach, he smiles shyly at the therapist and shows her his stuffed toy. He participates in play with the therapist after some prompting from his mother.

Ava, who had David when she was 21, has been his primary caretaker his entire life. They live with Ava's boyfriend in an apartment in a rough neighborhood—where David regularly hears gunshots and has seen people seriously injured. Three months ago, Ava was fired from her job at a call center. In the past few months, she has vacillated between withdrawal and irritability, which has resulted in far less positive reinforcement for her son. She has also been cutting her upper thigh with a razor in efforts to "feel something." She has harmed herself in the past, with the first instance occurring when she was a child. She tells the therapist that she works hard to be sure that David does not see her upset. Despite this, there have been times when she has unintentionally snapped at him. She tells the therapist, "I know he is just acting like a 4-year-old, but I get so frustrated."

From the age of 3 years, Ava was raised by her Aunt Lucille, who was a domestic worker. Ava's mother was unable to care for Ava because of a highly impairing substance use disorder, and her father was never part of her life. When Ava was 7 years old, Lucille's boyfriend moved into the home. A few months after moving in, he started abusing Lucille, both physically and emotionally. The abuse continued for the next 10 years. Ava's aunt was also raising one of her own children, and she had experienced homelessness in the past. Lucille could not cover the household bills on her own, and her boyfriend brought needed additional income. When he started abusing her, Lucille feared becoming homeless again if she left him.

Ava did well in school academically and generally performed at the top of her class. After her seventh-grade teacher noticed Ava's "attitude" and decreased engagement with her schoolwork, Ava was referred for mental health services. Although Lucille took Ava for her initial assessment, lapses in insurance coverage and inconsistent transportation prohibited regular follow-up. Per the clinic's policy, Ava was discharged after three no-shows.

David's therapist asks Ava to complete an ACE questionnaire for both herself and David, whose scores are 2 and 1, respectively. The case of Ava and David illustrates ways in which traumatic events and societal factors, including many that would not be adequately captured by typical psychiatric diagnostic schemes, contribute to the etiology and perpetuation of mental illness in individuals and across generations.

Multisystem Failure: Intergenerational Trauma, Financial Instability, and Food Insecurity

In the case example, Ava's unaddressed trauma symptoms were intruding not only on her internal life but also on her parenting. The financial insecurity in Ava's childhood home directly contributed to both her traumatic exposures and her inability to engage in treatment, even though there was early identification of a mental health problem. A generation later, following an exacerbation of her own symptoms, Ava found herself unemployed, a circumstance that has a demonstrated link to adverse mental health outcomes, particularly depression, suicidality, and alcohol use disorder. Parental unemployment also correlates to increased risk of child maltreatment (Patwardhan et al. 2017). However, employment, even when full time, does not reliably provide families with financial security.

In the United States, where women are the primary source of income or a co-earner for more than 50% of families with children, a significant contributor to economic instability during childhood is the gender wage gap. In 2018, the gender wage gap for full-time workers was 18%—meaning that women earned $0.82 for every $1.00 that men earned. This gap exists when comparing within racial and ethnic groups (e.g., white women earn less than white men, and Black women earn less than Black men). However, the full-time wage disparity between Black and Latinx women and white men is most striking; Black women earn $0.62 and Latinx women earn $0.55 for every $1.00 that a white man earns (Hegewisch and Tesfaselassie 2019). Many factors likely contribute to this wage gap, including educational attainment, type of employment, location of employment, and level of experience. When researchers control for these factors, the gap appears to lessen, but it remains (Blau and Kahn 2016), pointing to sexism and racism as a factor. Additionally, because discrimination does not exist solely in how employers pay women, and underrepresented minority women in particular, simply evaluating the numbers misses the bigger picture. By the time a woman enters the labor market, she has potentially been influenced by societal and family expectations of work-family balance and has dealt with subtle pushes away from more technical careers as well as discriminatory hiring practices. The combination of the gender pay gap and having a single income increases the economic hardships that single-mother households face in the United States; these households also are extremely vulnerable to poverty in the setting of job loss or even decreased hours.

Although many workers in the United States make minimum wage, they are not making a livable wage. In Los Angeles, for example, the minimum wage is $12 per hour; however, the calculated living wage for a single adult with one child is approximately $31 per hour (Glasmeier 2020). In this situation, despite working 40 hours per week, a single parent earning minimum wage is still at risk of not having enough money to pay for rent, utilities, and food. The chronic stress of living in an environment of financial insecurity has a significant impact on developing children who are dependent on caregivers to nourish them both physically and emotionally. Even if a child's caregivers work two low-wage jobs and manage to cover the bills, they may be preoccupied with the unrelenting urgency of feeding, clothing, and housing their children and may be less available to meet their child's psychological needs. *Secure attachment* provides a foundation for emotional regulation and distress tolerance, self-worth, and a sense of agency, and its development is threatened when caregivers cannot meet children's needs. In contrast, *insecure attachment* is a risk factor for emotional dysregulation, negative self-concept, and an external locus of control.

Children are navigating all of these stressors with immature brains that may be inadequately fueled for healthy neurocognitive growth. Food insecurity conveys increased risk for developmental delays, growth stunting, and inadequate cognitive development; it has been linked to poorer academic performance, absenteeism, and grade retention. Symptoms of ADHD, particularly hyperactivity and impulsivity, have also been linked to food insecurity. This relationship persists even after adjusting for individual and family characteristics, such as age of the child, race, ethnicity, household income, parental level of education, and parental mental health (Lu et al. 2019). Furthermore, after controlling for other aspects of socioeconomic status, food insecurity is associated with increased risk of mood, anxiety, behavior, and substance disorders in adolescents (McLaughlin et al. 2012). The resultant limitations in function reliably and predictably hamper upward mobility, trapping many individuals in intergenerational cycles of trauma and poverty. In David's case, three generations—he, his mother, and his mother's primary caretaker—were all impacted. Further exploration may reveal exposure even higher in the genogram. For Ava, David, and many others presenting to their pediatricians and mental health clinicians with "problem" behaviors, it is clear that early, chronic, inescapable traumatic exposure plays a significant role in the perpetuation of trauma and the manifestation of externalizing symptoms.

Professional Neglect of Structural and Complex Traumas

The diagnosis of PTSD was introduced in DSM-III in 1980 with criteria informed by symptoms that emerged in the context of a circumscribed, identifiable traumatic experience (e.g., exposure to war combat, rape) (American Psychiatric Association 1980). This was an important step in diagnostic psychiatric classification because it rooted psychological trauma symptoms in the precipitating stressor rather than individual weakness, as had been the case in previous DSM editions (Friedman 2019). However, the criteria for PTSD, in both previous and current DSM editions, fail to acknowledge traumas commonly experienced by children in marginalized communities. As a result, the psychological and physical impact of racism, oppression, and structural trauma too often is treated as an afterthought and relegated to a V code (ICD-10-CM codes for factors influencing health status and contact with health services), if considered at all (Cooper et al. 2008).

Complex PTSD (C-PTSD) is a potential consequence of exposure to these complex traumas, which occur over extended periods of time and from which the victim is unable to escape. First characterized by psychiatrist Judith Herman (1992), the conceptualization of complex trauma and the related diagnosis of C-PTSD provide a more patient-centered and trauma-informed approach for the diagnosis and treatment of patients such as David and Ava who have been exposed early in life to chronic, repetitive, harmful events that undermine safety, security, and healthy attachment. The captivity component of complex trauma is nearly universal in the traumatic experiences of children who have no power to remove themselves from their home or community environments. In addition to the three symptom clusters of PTSD (reexperiencing, avoidance, and sense of threat), C-PTSD includes three additional symptoms: affect dysregulation, negative concept of self, and difficulties in relationships (World Health Organization 2018). In 2018, C-PTSD was added to ICD-11 as a distinct entity from PTSD; the purpose was to more accurately reflect the pervasive psychological impact inflicted by complex trauma (Brewin et al. 2017). Although DSM-5 (American Psychiatric Association 2013) does not include C-PTSD, a new childhood diagnosis with irritabilty as a core symptom, disruptive mood dysregulation disorder (DMDD) was added. Notably, this diagnosis had far less empirical support than C-PTSD and does not mention trauma (Böttche et al. 2018; Roy et al. 2014).

In DSM-5, PTSD criteria have been added for children ages 6 years and younger, and the criteria for PTSD include new notes about diagnosing this disorder in adolescents and children older than 6 years. Although these additions represent an improvement, DSM-5 still fails to address the omission of the more chronic and pervasive traumatic experiences that affect many disenfranchised youth. In the case illustration, Ava could meet DSM-5 criterion A for PTSD because she directly witnessed physical violence toward her caregiver, yet David could not because his traumatic exposures occurred in his community. If DSM-5 criteria are dutifully applied, David's psychological symptoms stemming from his exposure to community violence, which occurred over time and at a critical developmental stage, may be misinterpreted. Additionally, in working with children, mental health professionals can find it challenging to elicit symptoms described in criteria B (reexperiencing), C (avoidance), and D (negative thoughts and feelings). Limitations in children's language may result in difficulties describing emotions or intrusive thoughts, and avoidance symptoms may be more nuanced because children have little choice in their surroundings. Criterion E, the remaining, most readily identified symptom category in working with children, is characterized by hypervigilance and irritability and therefore overlaps with DMDD and oppositional defiant disorder (ODD).

In DSM-5, criterion A for ODD includes "a pattern of angry/irritable mood, argumentative/defiant behavior, or vindictiveness lasting at least 6 months" (p. 462); again, there is no mention of trauma. The ODD diagnosis is liberally applied to chronically traumatized children, whereas, as noted earlier, the diagnosis of C-PTSD has yet to be included in DSM-5. DSM-5's approach is curious, given that the environmental risk factors for ODD mirror commonly occurring and widely understood sources of child trauma: familial psychopathology, maltreatment, neglect, caregiver disharmony, parental maladaptive behavior, exposure to interparental violence, parental alcoholism, divorce, and poverty (Boden et al. 2010; Lynskey et al. 1994; Marmorstein et al. 2009; Odgers et al. 2007).

Exposure to neighborhood violence has been linked to the development of several mental health disorders, including, by strength of association, PTSD, externalizing behaviors, and internalizing disorders such as depression and anxiety. The correlation between community violence exposure and mental health outcomes exists for both direct and indirect exposure and is strongest for victimization (Fowler et al. 2009). When a

clinician sees a child in the office who, like David, presents with externalizing symptoms, assessing the child only for direct trauma or violence in
the home may miss the presence and impact of neighborhood trauma.
Families like David's often face significant barriers to accessing mental
health care. It is lamentable that even when families overcome these barriers, precious opportunities for intervention during critical developmental
periods are often squandered by the mental health care system. When
mental health professionals do not take into account complex and structural traumas, they might misdiagnose children, which can have numerous,
substantial implications: failure to receive the appropriate mental health
treatments; decreased likelihood of appropriate caregiver understanding
and community support; unwarranted exposure to mood stabilizer and antipsychotic medication side effects; and increased likelihood of negative social outcomes, including school-related problems and incarceration.

When mental health professionals do not recognize the detrimental effects
of complex and structural trauma, they may miss the resulting symptoms alto-
gether or misattribute them to diagnoses of ADHD, ODD, DMDD, conduct
disorder (CD), or bipolar spectrum disorder. Notably, whereas Black and Latinx males are approximately 40% less likely than white males to be diagnosed
with ADHD (Baglivio et al. 2017), Black males are 40% more likely and
Black females are 54% more likely than their white counterparts to be diagnosed with CD (Bird et al. 2001; Braun et al. 2008). Although the reasons
for these differences are unclear, in diagnoses with significant comorbidity
and symptom overlap, children who are disproportionately exposed to
structural traumas in the larger society are disproportionately given more
stigmatizing diagnoses by mental health professionals.

Moreover, widespread professional failure to recognize the contributions of structural racism to the presentation and diagnoses of youth has
implications both within and beyond the clinic. When Black children present with behavioral and emotional dysregulation, often in the form of disruptive behaviors, they are more likely to be given a CD diagnosis and
referred to the juvenile justice system than are their white counterparts,
who are often diagnosed, appropriately in most cases, with mood disorders
or trauma and referred to mental health treatment (Bean et al. 2006; Bird
et al. 2001; Burris et al. 2011). The clinical approach to these behaviors in
Black children echoes the larger societal narrative of their inherent "bad-
ness." All too often, they are feared and treated punitively rather than protected and treated compassionately; after all, the reasoning goes, if they are
inherently bad and meet the criteria for ODD or DMDD, there is no need
to conduct a thorough exploration of potential traumatic etiologies. Far too
often, on contact with the mental health system, these children and families
do not have their race-based trauma or its impact on them even acknowl-

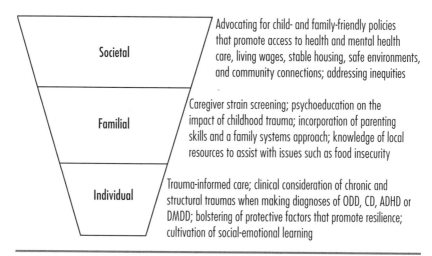

Societal — Advocating for child- and family-friendly policies that promote access to health and mental health care, living wages, stable housing, safe environments, and community connections; addressing inequities

Familial — Caregiver strain screening; psychoeducation on the impact of childhood trauma; incorporation of parenting skills and a family systems approach; knowledge of local resources to assist with issues such as food insecurity

Individual — Trauma-informed care; clinical consideration of chronic and structural traumas when making diagnoses of ODD, CD, ADHD or DMDD; bolstering of protective factors that promote resilience; cultivation of social-emotional learning

FIGURE 13–3. Potential interventions for childhood trauma.
Abbreviations. CD=conduct disorder; DMDD=disruptive mood dysregulation disorder; ODD=oppositional defiant disorder.
To view this figure in color, see Plate 4 in Color Gallery.

edged, let alone addressed. Without this acknowledgment, mental health professionals can perpetuate and inflict further trauma.

Interventions

Armed with knowledge of the structural determinants of health that disproportionately impact traumatized children and families, mental health clinicians are uniquely positioned not only to identify, diagnose, and treat trauma and complex trauma but also to advocate for children, patients, and communities. Interventions to address the issue of childhood trauma must occur at the societal, familial, and individual levels, as described in Figure 13–3. Of note, the pyramid is inverted as a visual representation of the child and family, who have relatively less power, bearing the weight of the upstream societal problems.

Progress in treating childhood trauma will require a significant paradigm shift within the mental health field, especially in the field of psychiatry—to view youth who need help not merely as biological and genetic entities with internal and external manifestations of psychopathology but as young human beings whose thoughts, feelings, and behaviors must be assessed and addressed in the context of where they live, learn, and play. Although psychosocial interventions to promote resilience and mental health interventions to address illness certainly have their place, true care for society's most vulnerable citizens demands structural shifts that prioritize children's safety, security, and opportunity.

Conclusion

"Denial, repression, and dissociation operate on a social as well as an individual level" (Herman 1992, p. 2). For clinicians, acknowledging the rampant existence of chronic childhood trauma is difficult. Acknowledging our role as citizens and clinician bystanders is even harder. A myopic focus on resilience is self-serving in that it places the onus for recovery on the traumatized, frequently underresourced child and family—and requires no change, discomfort, or hardship from the mental health field or society at large. History is repeating itself. Before PTSD was included in DSM-III, the trauma of rape victims and war veterans, for example, was not acknowledged in their diagnoses. Now, despite diagnostic changes to PTSD in DSM-5, we still give symptomatic, traumatized children diagnoses that do not acknowledge their trauma and, in the case of ODD and CD, diagnoses that are stigmatizing and curtail opportunities. Aided and abetted by the field of psychiatry, our broader society has, quite effectively, achieved a comfortable distance from the issue of children's chronic victimization. However, comfort and distance are luxuries that these children do not have. One could postulate that a problem of such reach and magnitude is not being readily acknowledged both because of the troubling reality it tells about our society and because of the status, or lack thereof, of its victims. Children have little power, and children who can be othered because of their race, class, or both have even less. A social justice framework demands that we, as knowledgeable mental health professionals and as privileged members of the larger society are impartial bystanders no more.

Questions for Self-Reflection

1. Which types of traumas do I tend to acknowledge or empathize with, and which types of traumas do I tend to overlook?
2. How might social injustice contribute to a PTSD diagnosis? How might social injustice contribute to a complex PTSD diagnosis?
3. As a clinician, administrator, or citizen, have I served in the role of bystander to the interpersonal trauma of children? To the structural trauma of children?

References

American Psychiatric Association: Diagnostic and Statistical Manual of Mental Disorders, 3rd Edition. Washington, DC, American Psychiatric Association, 1980

American Psychiatric Association: Diagnostic and Statistical Manual of Mental Disorders, 5th Edition. Arlington, VA, American Psychiatric Association, 2013

Asian American Federation: The State of Asian American Children. New York, Asian American Federation, 2014. Available at: http://www.aafederation.org/doc/AAF_StateofAsianAmericanChildren.pdf. Accessed May 12, 2020.

Baglivio MT, Wolff K, Piquero AR, et al: Racial/ethnic disproportionality in psychiatric diagnoses and treatment in a sample of serious juvenile offenders. J Youth Adolesc 46:1424–1451, 2017

Bean RA, Barber BK, Crane DR: Parental support, behavioral control, and psychological control among African American youth: the relationships to academic grades, delinquency, and depression. J Fam Issues 27:1335–1355, 2006

Benson PL: Developmental assets and asset-building community: conceptual and empirical foundations, in Developmental Assets and Asset-Building Communities: Implications for Research, Policy, and Practice. Edited by Lerner RM, Benson PL. New York, Kluwer Academic/Plenum, 2003, pp 19–43

Bird HR, Canino GJ, Davies M, et al: Prevalence and correlates of antisocial behaviors among three ethnic groups. J Abnorm Child Psychol 29:465–478, 2001

Blau FD, Kahn LM: The Gender Wage Gap: Extent, Trends, and Explanations. Working Paper No 21913. Cambridge, MA, National Bureau of Economic Research, 2016

Boden J, Ferguson D, Horwood LJ: Risk factors for conduct disorder and oppositional defiant disorder: evidence from a New Zealand birth cohort. J Am Acad Child Adolesc Psychiatry 49:1125–1133, 2010

Böttche M, Ehring T, Krüger-Gottschalk A, et al: Testing the ICD-11 proposal for complex PTSD in trauma-exposed adults: factor structure and symptom profiles. Eur J Psychotraumatol 9:1512264, 2018

Braun JM, Froehlich TE, Daniels JL, et al: Association of environmental toxicants and conduct disorder in U.S. children: NHANES 2001–2004. Environ Health Perspect 116:956–962, 2008

Brewin CR, Cloitre M, Hyland P, et al: A review of current evidence regarding the ICD-11 proposals for diagnosing PTSD and complex PTSD. Clin Psychol Rev 58:1–15, 2017

Burris FA, Breland-Noble AM, Webster JL, Soto JA: Juvenile mental health courts for adjudicated youth: role implications for child and adolescent psychiatric mental health nurses. J Child Adolesc Psychiatr Nurs 24:114–121, 2011

Carrion VG, Weems CF, Reiss RD, Ray AL: Towards an empirical definition of pediatric PTSD: the phenomenology of PTSD symptoms in youth. J Am Acad Child Adolesc Psychiatry 41:166–173, 2002

Centers for Disease Control and Prevention: About the CDC-Kaiser ACE Study. Atlanta, GA, Centers for Disease Control and Prevention, April 13, 2020. Available at: www.cdc.gov/violenceprevention/childabuseandneglect/acestudy/about.html. Accessed April 30, 2020.

Chen C, Burke Harris N: A Hidden Crisis: Findings on Adverse Childhood Experiences in California: Data Report. San Francisco, CA, Center for Youth Wellness, 2014

Cooper S, McLoyd V, Wood D, Hardaway C: Racial discrimination in the mental health of African-American adolescents, in Handbook of Race, Racism and the Developing Child. Edited by Quintana S, McKown C. Hoboken, NJ, Wiley, 2008, pp 278–312

Cronholm PF, Forke CM, Wade R, et al: Adverse childhood experiences: expanding the concept of adversity. Am J Prev Med 49:354–361, 2015

Cross D, Ruchard A, Jovanovic T, et al: Trauma exposure, PTSD, and parenting in a community sample of low income, predominantly African-American mothers and children. Psychol Trauma 10:327–335, 2018

DeBellis MD: Developmental traumatology: the psychobiological development of maltreated children and its implications for research, treatment, and policy. Dev Psychopathol 13:539–564, 2001

Edalati H, Nichols T, Crocker A, et al: Adverse childhood experiences in the risk of criminal justice involvement and victimization among homeless adults with mental illness. Psychiatr Serv 68:1288–1295, 2017

Felitti VJ, Anda RF, Nordenberg D, et al: Relationship of childhood abuse and household dysfunction to many of the leading causes of death in adults: the Adverse Childhood Experiences (ACE) Study. Am J Prev Med 14:245–258, 1998

Fowler PJ, Tompsett CJ, Braciszewski JM, et al: Community violence: a meta-analysis on the effect of exposure and mental health outcomes of children and adolescents. Dev Psychopathol 21:227–259, 2009

Friedman M: PTSD History and Overview. Washington, DC, U.S. Department of Veterans Affairs, October 14, 2019. Available at: www.ptsd.va.gov/professional/treat/essentials/history_ptsd.asp. Accessed January 3, 2020.

Glasmeier A: Living Wage Calculation for Los Angeles County, California. Cambridge, MA, Massachusetts Institute of Technology, 2020. Available at: https://livingwage.mit.edu/counties/06037. Accessed September 7, 2020.

Hegewisch A, Tesfaselassie A: The Gender Wage Gap: 2018; Earnings Differences by Gender, Race and Ethnicity. Washington, DC, Institute for Women's Policy Research, September 11, 2019. Available at https://iwpr.org/publications/annual-gender-wage-gap-2018. Accessed May 12, 2020.

Herman JL: Trauma and Recovery. New York, Basic Books, 1992

Lu S, Perez L, Leslein A, Hatsu I: The relationship between food insecurity and symptoms of attention-deficit hyperactivity disorder in children: a summary of the literature. Nutrients 11(3):659–671, 2019

Lynskey MT, Fergusson DM, Horwood LJ: The effect of parental alcohol problems on rates of adolescent psychiatric disorders. Addiction 89:1277–1286, 1994

Marmorstein NR, Iacono WG, McGue M: Alcohol and illicit drug dependence among parents: associations with offspring externalizing disorders. Psychol Med 39:149–155, 2009

McLaughlin KA, Green JG, Alegria M, et al: Food insecurity and mental disorders in a national sample of U.S. adolescents. J Am Acad Child Adolesc Psychiatry 51:1293–1303, 2012

Merrick MT, Ford DC, Ports KA, Guinn AS: Prevalence of adverse childhood experiences from the 2011–2014 Behavioral Risk Factor Surveillance System in 23 states. JAMA Pediatr 172:1038–1044, 2018

Mohammad E, Shapiro E, Wainwright L: Impacts of family and community violence exposure on child coping and mental health. J Abnorm Child Psychol 43(2):203–215, 2015

National Center for Children in Poverty: Child Poverty. New York, National Center for Children in Poverty, 2019. Available at: http://nccp.org/topics/childpoverty.html. Accessed January 3, 2020.

National Center for Education Statistics: Table 102.60, in Digest of Education Statistics. Washington, DC, National Center for Education Statistics, 2017. Available at: https://nces.ed.gov/programs/digest/d17/tables/dt17_102.60.asp?referer=raceindicators. Accessed May 12, 2020.

Odgers CL, Milne BJ, Caspi A, et al: Predicting prognosis for the conduct-problem boy: can family history help? J Am Acad Child Adolesc Psychiatry 46:1240–1249, 2007

Office of the Assistant Secretary for Planning and Evaluation: Poverty Guidelines. Washington, DC, U.S. Department of Health and Human Services, January 8, 2020. Available at: https://aspe.hhs.gov/poverty-guidelines. Accessed January 23, 2020.

Patwardhan I, Hurley KD, Thompson RW, et al: Child maltreatment as a function of cumulative family risk: findings from the Intensive Family Preservation Program. Child Abuse Negl 70:92–99, 2017

Roos L, Mota N, Afifi T, et al: Relationship between adverse childhood experiences and homelessness and the impact of Axis I and II disorders. Am J Public Health 103(suppl 2):S275–S281, 2013

Roy AK, Lopes V, Klein R: Disruptive mood dysregulation disorder (DMDD): a new diagnostic approach to chronic irritability in youth. Am J Psychiatry 171:918–924, 2014

Sabol WJ, Coulton CJ, Korbin JE: Building community capacity for violence prevention. J Interp Violence 19(3):322–340, 2004

Smith JR: Unequal burdens of Loss: Examining the frequency and timing of homicide deaths experienced by young black men across the life course. Am J Public Health 105:S483–S490, 2015

Solar O, Irwin A: A conceptual framework for action on the social determinants of health, in Social Determinants of Health, Discussion Paper 2 (Policy and Practice). Geneva, Switzerland, World Health Organization, 2010

Warnken H, Lauritsen JL: Who Experiences Victimization and Who Accesses Services? Findings from the National Crime Victimization Survey for Expanding Our Reach. Washington, DC, Office for Victims of Crime, 2019

World Health Organization: International Classification of Diseases, 11th Revision. Geneva, Switzerland, World Health Organization, 2018

PART IV

ACHIEVING MENTAL HEALTH EQUITY

CHAPTER 14

Social Justice and Mental Health System Reform

Phillip Murray, M.D., M.P.H.
Ruth S. Shim, M.D., M.P.H.

The current mental health care system in the United States both reflects and perpetuates the inequities evident in society. Fee-for-service, insurance-based health care models fuel a fragmented system that fails to incentivize population-based interventions or preventive measures. Broader, pervasive issues such as stigma and exposure to adverse social determinants of health can present barriers to treatment and precipitate or worsen psychiatric conditions. Less than half of people with a diagnosed mental health condition get treatment (Wang et al. 2002), and suicide rates have increased 35% within the past two decades, from an annual rate of 10.5 to 14.2 per 100,000 individuals (Hedegaard et al. 2020). The overall impact of mental health care is limited by little focus on mental illness prevention and by limited investment in interventions outside of direct clinical care. The structure of the U.S. health care system disproportionately burdens patients, larger communities, and seemingly unrelated safety net systems to attempt to pick up the slack with limited resources.

As health care professionals, we often idealize health care as a special field maintaining the highest standards of morality and humanism. Unfortunately, these ideals do not insulate either clinicians or patients from the faults of the health care system, especially in mental health. Transforming the mental health care system would require a reexamination of our core values and principles, particularly as they relate to how we define treatment; how we deliver services; and how we approach oppressed, underserved, and socially disadvantaged people. We might envision a mental health care system with patient-centered treatments, improved social services, and population-based public health interventions to address factors outside of health care that leave people vulnerable to psychiatric illnesses. This mental health care system would collaborate with other sectors to aid in recovery and would allow people to live meaningful lives, without barriers to accessing needed services. In this chapter, we outline prior mental health system reforms, factors that have led to difficulties within the current system, and future directions for successful reform.

What It Could Be: The Trieste Model of Mental Health Care

The public psychiatry model in Trieste, Italy, provides a vision of an effective, patient-centered mental health care system. The model, pioneered by Franco Basaglia in the 1970s, promotes the concept that the patient, not symptoms, are at the core of treatment (Mezzina 2014; Portacolone et al. 2015). This philosophical change has led to a system grounded in community-based treatment, with limited use of acute services. Treatment planning focuses on the creation of a meaningful and productive life. This is accomplished through a network of community mental health centers (CMHCs) that are open 24 hours a day, 7 days a week. Each center has a catchment area and is run by a multidisciplinary team from settings outside hospital environments.

The Trieste Department of Mental Health takes responsibility for the catchment area's mental health and social services, including supported housing and employment. The social and economic environment in Trieste prioritizes wellness and integration over cost savings. The program developers also highly value family cohesion and a core belief in the social inclusion of people with severe mental illnesses. Although acute care services are available, there is less focus on crisis stabilization and greater emphasis on social services that people need to thrive. This is reflected in the budget, which spends 94% on community services and 6% on acute services (Mezzina 2014; Portacolone et al. 2015). The model has been successful in cutting suicides and emergency department presentations in half and in reducing psychotic symptoms by 20% (Mezzina 2014). The Trieste model serves as a World Health Organization collaborating center, and the Department of Mental Health works to help other countries expand their community-based mental health services (World Health Organization 2020).

What It Was and What It Is Now: Present-Day Mental Health Care Reform

The current U.S. system is rooted in *deinstitutionalization*, a trend that started several decades ago, in which patients with mental illnesses were moved from state institutions to community settings (Goldman and Morrissey 1985). The Community Mental Health Centers Act of 1963 established CMHCs with the goal of providing integrated services in community settings (Goldman and Morrissey 1985). The location changed, but services were not bolstered enough to provide the appropriate support for people to thrive in the community. Without a comprehensive plan to address the complex needs of delivering care in the community, people with severe mental illnesses were shifted to other institutions, a practice termed *transinstitutionalization* (Mechanic and Grob 2006). The developing insurance-based health system was poorly equipped to address the needs of people with serious and persistent mental illnesses, resulting in significant inequities in coverage for mental health care compared with other health conditions.

Citing concerns regarding unnecessary spending, insurance companies provided minimal coverage with limited reimbursements for mental health care services at rates that were not comparable to those for other medical services. However, instead of controlling spending, lack of insurance parity further limited access to treatment by decreasing viable options for mental health coverage. Driven by profits, insurance companies had no incentive to change these policies without external regulation. The Mental Health Parity Act of 1996 attempted to address the issue by ensuring that lifetime expenditure caps for mental health services were equal to those for other medical conditions. The Mental and Health Parity and Addiction Equity Act of 2008 built on the Mental Health Parity Act by adding rules to increase equity in behavioral health coverage, reimbursements, and limits on care. Unfortunately, without a law mandating that insurance companies provide mental health coverage, many insurance companies opted to offer plans that did not cover any mental health services in order to avoid implementing parity requirements (Frank et al. 2014).

The 2010 Patient Protection and Affordable Care Act (ACA) further expanded health care coverage through the individual mandate and Medicaid expansion and, importantly, categorized mental health and substance use disorder services as essential health benefits. In addition to providing coverage for people with limited income, Medicaid also pays for specialized services for individuals with disabilities, including supported employment programs and some case coordination. Legal challenges to the ACA led to a 2012 U.S. Supreme Court ruling that made Medicaid expansion optional for states, and several governors opposed expansion for reasons ranging from the belief that Medicaid did more harm than good to concerns that entitlement programs such as Medicaid create dependency (Sommers and Epstein 2013). However, in a systematic review of Medicaid expansion under the ACA, Mazurenko et al. (2018) found increases in coverage, service use, and quality of care, and very few studies reported any negative consequences.

Where It Needs to Go: Recommendations and Rationale for Reform

If our aim is to transform the U.S. mental health care system into a patient-centered, population-based system focused on equitable outcomes and the promotion of mental health, rather than a system focused on symptom and crisis management, we must consider a multifactorial approach balancing immediate and long-term changes. Recommendations to reform the U.S. mental health care system include improving access to mental health care services, building the mental health workforce, and restructuring mental health care service delivery. Unfortunately, multiple stakeholders who hold power have various vested interests in keeping mental health care services fragmented and dysfunctional. Transforming this system will come about not as a result of goodwill or sudden enlightenment but rather from directed advocacy and coordination of a range of stakeholders dedicated to minimizing the unacceptable outcomes that currently plague our mental health care system.

Improve Access to Mental Health Care Services

Universal Health Care

A single-payer, universal health care system would eliminate many of the conflicting interests within the health system, including prioritizing profits over people. A single entity would have less incentive to focus on individual health care procedures and would emphasize the outcomes of interventions. Streamlining services would decrease inefficiencies and repetition that come from working in silos, thus saving on administrative costs. Additionally, universal health care would significantly and almost immediately benefit people with serious mental illnesses by providing health insurance benefits to individuals who often have barriers in securing the types of jobs that are typically associated with health insurance in the United States.

The current system is plagued with philosophical and practical deficits, and making a transition to a single-payer system seems like an insurmountable task. Despite the barriers, if the goal is to reduce inequities and injustice within mental health, then it is perhaps the most critical aspiration to strive for. However, until such a transition occurs, we can take more incremental steps to improve the current mental health care system.

Medicaid Expansion

Medicaid expansion in all states provides a viable path for increased access to mental health care services. In a comparison of those states that expanded Medicaid to those states that did not, several patterns emerge (Guth et al. 2020). Expansion states saw a decrease in their uninsured population among low-income individuals, rural residents, and other vulnerable populations in most racial and ethnic categories, and these populations had increased access to behavioral health and substance use disorder services. Instead of experiencing an increased financial burden, those states that expanded Medicaid services observed increased cost savings, decreased burdens for uncompensated care, and decreased costs per Medicaid enrollee. Medicaid expansion also demonstrated improvements in enrollees' ability to continue work; decreased enrollees' out-of-pocket spending; and decreased poverty by 1% across Medicaid expansion states, representing 690,000 fewer Americans living in poverty (Zewde and Wirner 2019).

Despite the overwhelmingly positive evidence, some states still have not expanded Medicaid. Also, constant threats to the integrity of Medicaid exist at the federal and state levels, including efforts to add work requirements to Medicaid eligibility, which would create unnecessary barriers to treatment access and likely fuel circumstances that lead people to require more government assistance. Misplaced ideas of autonomy and dependency on entitlement programs continue to hinder necessary progress for vulnerable populations. As described in previous chapters, these poor outcomes are the result of structural-level barriers, and therefore the solutions require structural rather than individual interventions. Stringent work requirements and reductions in social services ignore the lessons contained in the historical context that enabled the formation of a broken mental health care system in the first place. Without a historical perspective, these unrealistic expectations are, at best, misguided attempts at fostering autonomy and, at worst, punitive measures to prevent oppressed and vulnerable people from improving their status in life.

Build the Mental Health Workforce

Health Professional Shortage Areas

Even individuals with Medicaid coverage have challenges in accessing mental health care services. An estimated 2.5 million Medicaid enrollees had unmet mental health needs in 2015 (Zur et al. 2017). These unmet mental health needs are partially the result of a shortage of mental health professionals (e.g., psychiatrists, psychologists, clinical social workers, psychiatric nurses, marriage and family therapists, licensed professional counselors, peer support workers) and the fact that few psychiatrists in private practices accept Medicaid as payment (Bishop et al. 2014). Health Professional Shortage Areas (HPSAs) are designated areas that have shortages in any of three health care categories: primary medical care, dental care, and mental health care (Kaiser Family Foundation 2019). Mental health care HPSAs are designated as areas with less than one mental health professional per 30,000 people. The United States currently has more than 6,000 mental health care HPSAs, accounting for nearly 113 million people—fully one-third of the population (Kaiser Family Foundation 2019). Inadequate access to mental health care is further complicated by limited numbers of mental health professionals in rural areas and from racially and ethnically underrepresented backgrounds.

The National Health Service Corps (NHSC) was created to address HPSAs by paying up front for training programs with a guaranteed year-for-year repayment or loan repayment for yearly obligations to practice in HPSAs (U.S. Department of Health and Human Services 2017). Compared with the national workforce, the NHSC has had success recruiting a higher percentage of Black and Latinx physicians (U.S. Department of Health and Human Services 2017). Also, studies have demonstrated that compared with graduates from majority backgrounds, these graduates are more likely to work with underserved populations (Garcia et al. 2018). This program should be supported and expanded.

For individuals fortunate enough to have insurance coverage and live in areas with adequate numbers of mental health professionals, access to timely mental health care is still not a given. Psychiatrists have lower participation in health insurance networks compared with all other medical specialties, leading to the use of out-of-network benefits at higher rates, resulting in an increased financial burden for patients (Bishop et al. 2014; Cummings et al. 2013). Insurance companies often supply outdated lists of available mental health professionals, further complicating and prolonging the referral process. These barriers lead to long wait times for appointments, averaging approximately 1 month for new adult outpatient appointments (Malowney et al. 2015). For children and adolescents, the wait time for a new outpatient appointment ranges from 30 to 50 days past wait times for general pediatrics appointments (Cama et al. 2017; Steinman et al. 2015). During this critical time, symptoms can worsen, leading to loss of functioning and missed school or work days and ultimately requiring higher levels of care.

For individuals in acute crises, there are approximately 11 inpatient psychiatric beds per 100,000 people. Three times more beds are needed for an adequate supply (Torrey et al. 2012). The average wait time for people in crisis to start treatment in an inpatient psychiatric facility is 3 days—or longer for certain populations, including children with special needs and autism spectrum diagnoses (La et al. 2015). During this time, people are held in medical facilities that are ill equipped to deal with active mental health crises. Although this situation would be unacceptable for most physical health conditions or acute injuries, this poor quality of care is accepted as the status quo for psychiatric emergencies.

Pipeline Programs

Within the mental health workforce, 6.2% of psychologists, 5.6% of advanced practice nurses, and 12.6% of social workers are from racial and ethnic minority backgrounds (Hoge et al. 2013). It is difficult to pinpoint exactly the number of psychiatrists from backgrounds that are underrepresented in medicine (URM), but figures from medical school matriculants indicate that this number is far lower than what is needed. Despite an increase in applications to medical school, URM female matriculants continue to be underrepresented by nearly 40% and URM male matriculants by close to 50% (Lett et al. 2019). The legacy of structural racism, both in society and in the field of medicine, contributes significantly to this underrepresentation. An important step toward dismantling the pernicious effects of structural racism is to undo subtle discriminatory policies that serve to exclude people from URM backgrounds from matriculating at and graduating from medical schools.

An important route to increasing URM representation in psychiatry is through pipeline programs that clear a more direct pathway to the field of medicine (Council on Graduate Medical Education 2005). Pipeline programs that begin early in young people's educational experiences can have the greatest impact. URM high school students exposed to science and mental health education programs may have their interest piqued, and doors that previously seemed closed can be opened. Undergraduate and postbaccalaureate programs can provide significant support for URM students with interests in psychiatry, psychology, or clinical social work. The American Psychiatric Association's Black Men in Psychiatry Early Pipeline Program specifically recruits Black male undergraduate students, increases their exposure to mentors in psychiatry, and provides support to foster success in medical school (American Psychiatric Association 2020).

Within medical schools, students from diverse backgrounds who have an interest in working with underserved or oppressed populations should be actively recruited to consider careers in psychiatry. Traditionally, many URM students have opted for primary care careers or other medical specialty fields that they feel maximize their effectiveness and impact on improving inequities in their local communities. However, it should be made clear to students of diverse backgrounds that their work to address the needs of vulnerable and oppressed communities can be effectively accomplished through careers in psychiatry. Medical education that emphasizes mental health equity, structural competence, and cultural humility is a critical part of the recruitment process (Rao et al. 2018).

Restructure Mental Health Service Delivery

Collaborative Care Models

As a result of the severe shortage of mental health care providers, psychiatric care services are more likely to be delivered in primary care settings than in specialty mental health care settings (Wang et al. 2005). The collaborative care approach was developed specifically to systematize the treatment of people with mild to moderate mental health and substance use problems that can be effectively managed in primary care with a stepped care approach. The model offers primary care providers decision-making support, treatment plan supervision, short-term consultation, and, if needed, referrals to specialty mental health care providers (Druss and Goldman 2018). The model allows mental health professionals to leverage their expertise using a population-based approach that successfully expands access to care.

Although the model is effective, the transition to collaborative care can represent a significant culture shift for many primary care practitioners. Financing collaborative care services can be challenging because states and insurance companies have adopted existing billing codes and payments at variable rates. Furthermore, mental health workforce shortages also impact collaborative care models. Identifying mental health professionals who are comfortable practicing in this model can be challenging because many are not specifically trained to deliver care in this way. Improving training to adequately prepare mental health professionals to work in collaborative care settings is an important step forward.

Social Determinants of Mental Health

Efforts to strengthen the mental health workforce will not necessarily guarantee quality care. The social determinants of mental health often contribute to poor mental health outcomes and drive mental health inequities (Compton and Shim 2015). For example, adverse childhood experiences are associated with mood and anxiety disorders, substance use disorders, and many behavioral risk factors for chronic disease, including early initiation of smoking and sexual activity (Mersky et al. 2013). Mental health and substance use disorders make up the majority of conditions that necessitate emergency department visits by homeless individuals (Wadhera et al. 2019). Income inequality is a factor in first admissions to psychiatric hospitalizations (Suokas et al. 2020), and people with lower socioeconomic status have higher rates of diagnoses of schizophrenia and major depressive disorder (Saraceno et al. 2005). Health systems, armed with these data, are beginning to operationalize taking action to address social determinants in clinical care, in part by making significant investments in support for housing, employment, education, food, and transportation (Horwitz et al. 2020). Ultimately, to improve the health and mental health of the U.S. population, mental health professionals should support policies that strengthen local and national social and public health services, which have a greater impact on improving health outcomes than spending invested in health care services (Bradley et al. 2016).

As racism and discrimination continue to be primary drivers of health care inequities, action to dismantle the dangerous effects of structural and interpersonal oppression is necessary to make any significant progress toward an equitable mental health care system. On a larger scale, decision makers in clinical care settings should commit to hiring staff who reflect the populations they are serving. Health systems and hospitals have the potential to function as anchor institutions, purposefully investing in, partnering with, and engaging more deeply and meaningfully with their local communities to improve neighborhood-level health outcomes (Koh et al. 2020).

Value-Based Payment Models

The current fee-for-service system incentivizes hospitals to focus on specialties that are reimbursed at much higher rates and allows insurance companies to limit the amount of care they pay for. Mental health services have been reimbursed at lower rates than other medical specialties, and caps have been placed on the number of services and therapy sessions provided in the name of profit (Frank et al. 2014). Low reimbursements discourage the much-needed investment in mental health services to address core factors that drive negative outcomes but do not contribute directly to the bottom line.

A solution to these challenges involves moving the system away from fee-for-service models and toward value-based models. One such model that moves the health system in this direction is the accountable care organization (ACO), which comprises a group of hospitals, physicians, and other health care providers coordinating care for a specific population of patients (Centers for Medicare and Medicaid Services 2020). Originally developed for Medicare enrollees, ACOs have successfully expanded to focus on other patient populations, and preliminary research has demonstrated that this model can also be successful for underserved or vulnerable patient populations. For example, states that participated in Medicaid expansion have applied the ACO model to their vulnerable patients (Mahadevan and Houston 2015), and individual systems have applied it to some of their highest utilizers of care. Core principles of success pertain to up-front funding, partnering with community organizations, and information sharing between different parts of the organization to ensure the best possible results.

After implementing ACO models across the state, Oregon has decreased inequities in primary care visits by Black and Indigenous patients in comparison to white patients (Mahadevan and Houston 2015). A recent meta-analysis also shows that ACOs have decreased the rate of potentially preventable hospitalizations for depressed patients with chronic conditions (Barath et al. 2020). Since the passage of the ACA, there are more than 500 Medicaid-specific ACOs that are impacting approximately 10 million lives (Castellucci 2020). Programs continue to have challenges with initial investments, and federal government divestment has led to decreased numbers of ACOs. However, transitioning from fee-for-service to value-based payment models is key to improving outcomes for people with mental illnesses and substance use disorders. Funding should be secured and systems should be supported to help drive the health care system in this direction.

Community-Partnered Participatory Research

Solutions to address the mental health consequences of social injustice will have to come from collaborations that leverage the expertise of health care institutions and community stakeholders. Community-partnered participatory research (CPPR) provides a framework for community program development and collaborative research to develop and implement solutions (Jones and Wells 2007). A key component of CPPR is equal power sharing between communities and academic institutions from the very beginning when issues are being identified (Jones and Wells 2007), in contrast to standard arrangements in which health systems and researchers have disproportionate control. This partnership continues throughout the subsequent steps of aligning resources, engaging and educating community members, and evaluating progress. Information is shared freely, and there is full transparency throughout the process (Jones and Wells 2007). CPPR differs from traditional research approaches in which academic institutions are at risk of exploiting community members under the auspices of gathering data, without accounting for or acknowledging power differentials or conflicting priorities. The CPPR approach requires a culture shift and more upfront investment in relationships and coalition building. This requires significant time but results in sustainable improvements for underresourced communities.

Community Partners in Care (CPIC) provides a glimpse of the CPPR model at work. CPIC implemented a quality improvement program for depression treatment in underresourced communities in Los Angeles (Wells et al. 2013). As compared with usual care, community engagement and planning led to significantly improved outcomes, including increased outpatient visits for depression care, increased physical activity, fewer risk factors for homelessness, and improved mental health and quality of life (Wells et al. 2013).

The successful adoption of CPPR models could be a path forward for CMHCs. Principles of coalition building through CPPR could help CMHCs prioritize community needs and develop and implement interventions to improve access to and quality of mental health care. The vision of what CMHCs could be in the United States has never been realized, but CPPR could help to move toward this ideal.

Conclusion

The current U.S. mental health care system is a reflection of a society that has not, to this point, placed value on the importance of preventing mental illness, promoting mental health, or reducing mental health inequities. Mental health care system reform must balance the urgency of improving a system that is failing most with the sheer magnitude of incremental changes needed to ensure that the system works well for all. Advocacy must simultaneously focus on realistic, incremental changes without losing sight of the ultimate goal of transformation into an equitable health care system. Solutions exist; therefore, we as health care professionals must not be complicit in accepting the social injustice that pervades our current mental health care system. We must advocate for a more just system that ensures that everyone has an equal opportunity to live with good mental health.

Questions for Self-Reflection

1. What is my stance on incremental versus radical mental health care system reform?
2. What reforms do I think are most necessary for the mental health care system to produce more equitable results?
3. What role might I play in advancing policies (both local and national) that are informed by principles of justice?

References

American Psychiatric Association: Black Men in Psychiatry. Washington, DC, American Psychiatric Association, 2020. Available at: www.psychiatry.org/residents-medical-students/medical-students/medical-student-programs/workforce-inclusion-pipeline/black-men-in-psychiatry. Accessed April 23, 2020.

Barath D, Amaize A, Chen J: Accountable care organizations and preventable hospitalizations among patienets with depression. Am J Prev Med 59(1):e1–e10, 2020

Bishop TF, Press MJ, Keyhani S, Pincus HA: Acceptance of insurance by psychiatrists and the implications for access to mental health care. JAMA Psychiatry 71:176–181, 2014

Bradley EH, Canavan M, Rogan E, et al: Variation in health outcomes: the role of spending on social services, public health, and health care, 2000–09. Health Aff 35:760–768, 2016

Cama S, Malowney M, Smith AJB, et al: Availability of outpatient mental health care by pediatricians and child psychiatrists in five U.S. cities. Int J Health Serv 47:621–635, 2017

Castellucci M: Participants continue to drop out of Medicare ACO program. Modern Healthcare, January 10, 2020. Available at: www.modernhealthcare.com/government/participants-continue-drop-out-medicare-aco-program. Accessed February 20, 2020.

Centers for Medicare and Medicaid Services: Accountable Care Organizations: General Information. Washington, DC, Centers for Medicare and Medicaid Services, February 25, 2020. Available at: https://innovation.cms.gov/initiatives/ACO. Accessed May 3, 2020.

Compton MT, Shim RS (eds): The Social Determinants of Mental Health. Washington, DC, American Psychiatric Association Publishing, 2015

Council on Graduate Medical Education: Sixteenth Report: Physician Workforce Policy Guidelines for the United States. Rockville, MD, Health Resources and Services Administration, 2005

Cummings JR, Wen H, Ko M, Druss BG: Geography and the Medicaid mental health care infrastructure: implications for health care reform. JAMA Psychiatry 70:1084–1090, 2013

Druss BG, Goldman HH: Integrating health and mental health services: a past and future history. Am J Psychiatry 175:1199–1204, 2018

Frank RG, Beronio K, Glied SA: Behavioral health parity and the Affordable Care Act. J Soc Work Disabil Rehabil 13:31–43, 2014

Garcia AN, Kuo T, Arangua L, Pérez-Stable EJ: Factors associated with medical school graduates' intention to work with underserved populations: policy implications for advancing workforce diversity. Acad Med 93:82–89, 2018

Goldman HH, Morrissey JP: The alchemy of mental health policy: homelessness and the fourth cycle of reform. Am J Public Health 75:727–731, 1985

Guth M, Garfield R, Rudowitz R: The Effects of Medicaid Expansion Under the ACA: Updated Findings From a Literature Review. San Francisco, CA, Kaiser Family Foundation, March 17, 2020. Available at: www.kff.org/medicaid/report/the-effects-of-medicaid-expansion-under-the-aca-updated-findings-from-a-literature-review. Accessed May 2, 2020.

Hedegaard H, Curtin S, Warner M: Increase in Suicide Mortality in the United States, 1999–2018. NCHS Data Brief No 362, April 2020. Atlanta, GA, Centers for Disease Control and Prevention, 2020

Hoge M, Stuart G, Morris J, et al: Mental health and addiction workforce development: federal leadership is needed to address the growing crisis. Health Aff 32:2005–2012, 2013

Horwitz LI, Chang C, Arcilla HN, Knickman JR: Quantifying health systems' investment in social determinants of health, by sector, 2017–19: study analyzes the extent to which U.S. health systems are directly investing in community programs to address social determinants of health. Health Aff 39:192–198, 2020

Jones L, Wells K: Strategies for academic and clinician engagement in community-participatory partnered research. JAMA 297:407–410, 2007

Kaiser Family Foundation: Mental Health Care Health Professional Shortage Areas. San Francisco, CA, Kaiser Family Foundation, September 30, 2019. Available at: www.kff.org/3bfeb38. Accessed February 20, 2020.

Koh HK, Bantham A, Geller AC, et al: Anchor institutions: best practices to address social needs and social determinants of health. Am J Public Health 110:309–316, 2020

La EM, Lich KH, Wells R, et al: Increasing access to state psychiatric hospital beds: exploring supply side solutions. Psychiatr Serv 67(5):523–528, 2015

Lett LA, Murdock HM, Orji WU, et al: Trends in racial/ethnic representation among U.S. medical students. JAMA Netw Open 2(9), e1910490, 2019

Mahadevan R, Houston R: Supporting social service delivery through Medicaid accountable care organizations: early state efforts. Hamilton, NJ, Center for Health Care Strategies, February 2015. Available at: www.chcs.org/media/Supporting-Social-Service-Delivery-Final_0212151.pdf. Accessed February 20, 2020.

Malowney M, Keltz S, Fischer D, Boyd JW: Availability of outpatient care from psychiatrists: a simulated-patient study in three U.S. cities. Psychiatr Serv 66:94–96, 2015

Mazurenko O, Balio CP, Agarwal R, et al: The effects of Medicaid expansion under the ACA: a systematic review. Health Aff 37:944–950, 2018

Mechanic D, Grob GN: Rhetoric, realities, and the plight of the mentally ill in America, in History and Health Policy in the United States: Putting the Past Back In. Edited by Stevens RA, Rosenberg CE, Burns LR. New Brunswick, NJ, Rutgers University Press, 2006, pp 229–249

Mersky JP, Topitzes J, Reynolds AJ: Impacts of adverse childhood experiences on health, mental health, and substance use in early adulthood: a cohort study of an urban, minority sample in the U.S. Child Abuse Negl 37:917–925, 2013

Mezzina R: Community mental health care in Trieste and beyond: an "open door-no restraint" system of care for recovery and citizenship. J Nerv Ment Dis 202:440–445, 2014

Portacolone E, Segal S, Mezzina R, et al: A tale of two cities: the exploration of the Trieste public psychiatry model in San Francisco. Cult Med Psychiatry 39:680–697, 2015

Rao S, How PC, Ton H: Education, training, and recruitment of a diverse workforce in psychiatry. Psychiatr Ann 48:143–148, 2018

Saraceno B, Levav I, Kohn R: The public mental health significance of research on socio-economic factors in schizophrenia and major depression. World Psychiatry 4:181–185, 2005

Sommers BD, Epstein AM: U.S. governors and the Medicaid expansion—no quick resolution in sight. N Engl J Med 368:496–499, 2013

Steinman KJ, Shoben AB, Dembe AE, Kelleher KJ: How long do adolescents wait for psychiatry appointments? Community Ment Health J 51:782–789, 2015

Suokas K, Koivisto A, Hakulinen C, et al: Association of income with the incidence rates of first psychiatric hospital admissions in Finland, 1996–2014. JAMA Psychiatry 77:274–284, 2020

Torrey EF, Fuller DA, Geller J, et al: No Room at the Inn: Trends and Consequences of Closing Public Psychiatric Hospitals. Arlington, VA, Treatment Advocacy Center, 2012

U.S. Department of Health and Human Services: National Health Service Corps Report to Congress for the Year 2016. Washington, DC, Health Resources and Services Administration, 2017. Available at: www.hrsa.gov/sites/default/files/hrsa/about/organization/bureaus/bhw/reportstocongress/2016-nhsc-rtc.pdf. Accessed February 20, 2020.

Wadhera RK, Choi E, Shen C, et al: Trends, causes, and outcomes of hospitalizations for homeless individuals: a retrospective cohort study. Med Care 57:21–27, 2019

Wang PS, Demler O, Kessler RC: Adequacy of treatment for serious mental illness in the United States. Am J Public Health 92:92–98, 2002

Wang PS, Lane M, Olfson M, et al: Twelve-month use of mental health services in the United States: results from the National Comorbidity Survey Replication. Arch Gen Psychiatry 62:629–640, 2005

Wells KB, Jones L, Chung B, et al: Community-partnered cluster-randomized comparative effectiveness trial of community engagement and planning or resources for services to address depression disparities. J Gen Intern Med 28:1268–1278, 2013

World Health Organization: WHO Collaborating Centre for Research and Training in Mental Health. Geneva, Switzerland, World Health Organization, 2020. Available at: www.euro.who.int/en/health-topics/noncommunicable-diseases/mental-health/partners/who-collaborating-centres-working-in-mental-health/who-collaborating-centre-for-research-and-training-in-mental-health. Accessed February 20, 2020.

Zewde N, Wirner C: Antipoverty impact of Medicaid growing with state expansions over time. Health Aff 38:132–138, 2019

Zur J, Musumeci MB, Garfield R: Medicaid's Role in Financing Behavioral Health Services for Low-Income Individuals. Menlo Park, CA, Kaiser Family Foundation, 2017

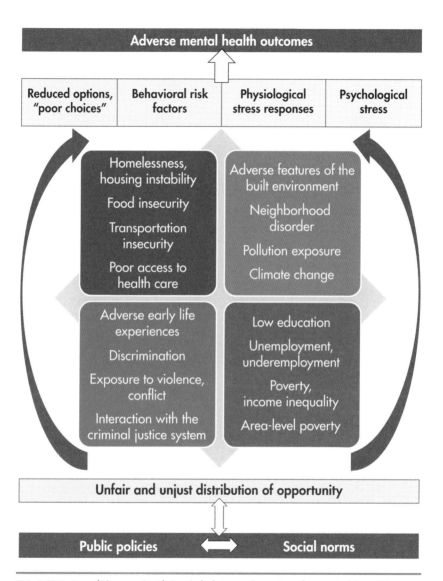

PLATE 1. *(Figure 2–1)* Social determinants of mental health framework.

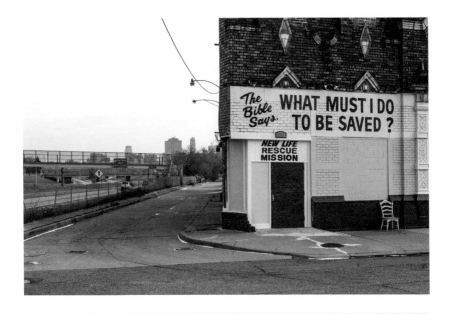

PLATE 2. *(Figure 7–1)* The Fisher Freeway, one example of the many interstates cutting through Detroit.

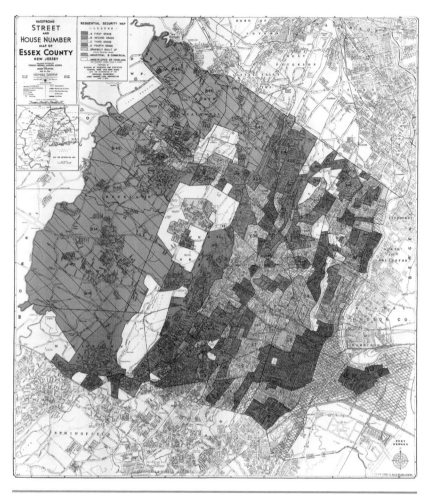

PLATE 3. *(Figure 7–2)* Residential security map of Essex County, New Jersey.

Source. Courtesy of the National Archives, Washington, DC.

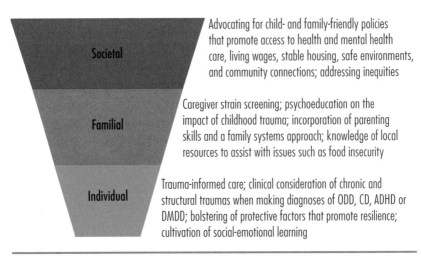

Societal — Advocating for child- and family-friendly policies that promote access to health and mental health care, living wages, stable housing, safe environments, and community connections; addressing inequities

Familial — Caregiver strain screening; psychoeducation on the impact of childhood trauma; incorporation of parenting skills and a family systems approach; knowledge of local resources to assist with issues such as food insecurity

Individual — Trauma-informed care; clinical consideration of chronic and structural traumas when making diagnoses of ODD, CD, ADHD or DMDD; bolstering of protective factors that promote resilience; cultivation of social-emotional learning

PLATE 4. *(Figure 13–3)* Potential interventions for childhood trauma.

Abbreviations. CD=conduct disorder; DMDD=disruptive mood dysregulation disorder; ODD=oppositional defiant disorder.

CHAPTER 15

Social Justice and Advocacy

Kali D. Cyrus, M.D., M.P.H.
Sarah Y. Vinson, M.D.

Advocacy takes, and is needed in, many forms, yet our level of engagement in advocacy as mental health professionals often falls short. As clinicians, we are charged with supporting patients' progress toward recovery even when much of what makes them sick or well cannot be addressed by our staying in our proverbial lane. When distress and functional impairment are driven by our patients' experiences of oppression, criteria-based diagnostic and treatment approaches are merely a symptomatic intervention. In true patient-centered care, the patient is viewed in the context of cultural, societal, and structural factors that drive mental health outcomes. Who among us with a chronic bacterial infection wreaking havoc on our bodies would opt for purely symptomatic treatment? Although the use of pain relievers might ease our discomfort, they would have no power to restore us to health. We would want, perhaps even demand, antibiotics as the best opportunity for a cure. As mental health professionals, we have ethical duties of beneficence and nonmaleficence, and the perpetual focus on symptom alleviation is an abdication of our professional responsibilities.

Simply put, for oppressed people, advocacy is required for true recovery. Although it is true that in most cases, the complete restoration of justice is far beyond our ability, it is also true that in most cases, furthering justice—in some way—is well within our reach.

Advocacy is necessary, but it is not easy. And we know it. Most health care providers recognize advocacy's importance but doubt their ability to even influence their own health care system (The Physicians Foundation 2018). The problems posed by oppression are big, complex, and entrenched in every societal system, and we are individuals, with limited knowledge, who can feel lost about where to start. That said, we have all done hard things before. No one is merely handed professional degrees, graduate degrees, professional licenses, or board certifications. These credentials are earned by highly capable, highly motivated people with a desire to serve. Like clinical skills, advocacy skills can be learned and put into practice. As described in this chapter, this endeavor can be approached through a three-part strategy: 1) develop a new knowledge base, 2) recognize injustice and your role in addressing it, and 3) respond to injustice through an iterative, sustainable process.

Develop a New Knowledge Base

As highly trained, skilled clinicians, mental health professionals have true expertise. This expertise, however, often does not extend to advocacy. Our schooling process grounds us in theories of psychology and the understanding of countertransference but provides little education in systems of inequity or in examining our engagement with them. Much like the diligence required to identify clinical pearls for treatment, diligence is required to identify the manifestations of injustice for advocacy (Stege et al. 2017). Because of the myriad manifestations of oppressive dynamics, basic understanding starts with an interdisciplinary knowledge base. The lens through which this information is sought, filtered, and received is critical, meaning clinician-advocates must also build self-awareness. Thus, building foundational knowledge for advocacy is a two-part process—a study of self and a study of systems.

Mental health professionals are people. People are biased. This bias is shaped by people's experiences within their families and the broader society. Inequity permeates every American system, and our educational and training systems are no exception. Despite the many years of training required to earn professional credentials, there is still a great deal to learn to support people with mental illnesses and substance use disorders in their healing and recovery. For mental health professionals who have invested tremendous money, time, and effort into their clinical training, and who may also hold some measure of personal value in their professional identities, acknowledging inequity and its implications can be personally challenging.

For you as a mental health professional, the willingness to assess your position of power relative to others is critical, but doing so may arouse shame, guilt, and insecurity (Chung et al. 2018). If you were raised in a nice suburb of a major city, you were the beneficiary of redlining (a concept discussed in Chapter 7, "Social Injustice and Urban Development"). If you attended good schools during your primary educational process, you had a marked advantage over those who did not. If you smoked marijuana but were never searched because you did not look like an *addict*, your actions were no different from those that resulted in the criminalization and disenfranchisement of many Americans. It is natural to allay or, when possible, entirely avoid discomfort, and it follows that working to understand your privilege may activate defenses. Self-reflection and curiosity are needed to recognize when this defensiveness occurs, and humility and commitment are needed to manage discomfort and defenses and then to persist.

A practical approach to beginning advocacy is to explore our individual identities, the social status of the groups to which we belong, and their salience to us. Table 15–1 provides three illustrations of this process.

The study of systems and theories should be guided by individual interests and learning styles. Additionally, patient populations served should inform the study content. For example, a counselor who works in a federally qualified health center in Ferguson, Missouri, should become educated about the gross inequities in the local criminal justice system that preceded the 2014 killing of Michael Brown and the following protests. A child psychiatrist who works in group homes should explore the structural traumas exacted by the child welfare system. And a forensic psychologist consulting to courts should examine the bias inherent in so-called objective testing results. Much content and knowledge of structures and systems can be gained through literature, podcasts, or even documentaries (see Chapter 16, "Social Justice and Mental Health: A Call to Action" for a preliminary list). Dialogue is another important process for understanding oppression, power, and privilege and for stimulating awareness. Dialogue requires mutual respect between participants, compassion in listening and responding, and value for the resulting generation of new knowledge (Hunt et al. 2019). Regardless of the learning process used, increased knowledge of social injustice and decreased defensiveness to acknowledging it are foundational elements of advocacy.

TABLE 15–1. Examples of power, individual identity, and group membership salience in clinicians

Consider descriptions of three mental health professionals and advocates from different social groups, with varying levels of membership salience and their hypothetical perceptions of power:

	Clinician 1	Clinician 2	Clinician 3
Career stage	Early career	Midcareer	Senior
Race	Asian and white (biracial)	Black	White
Appearance	Pale skin, dark hair	Dark skin, dark hair	Olive skin, light hair
Ethnicity	Vietnamese American	Non-Hispanic	Eastern European
Family history	Father is second generation born in United States, and grandparents immigrated shortly after the Vietnam War	Does not know historical background of enslaved ancestors, but grandparents were free	First generation born in United States; grandparents were Holocaust survivors
Sexuality	Queer Came out of the closet after college, so most of social network is heterosexual	Asexual Open to romantic connections but not interested in sexual relationships	Heterosexual
Relationship status	In a relationship	Single	Married to high school sweetheart
Gender identity	Cisgender female (she/her/hers) Born biological female; appearance is androgynous, with stereotypically masculine dress style	Genderqueer (they/their/ theirs) Born biological female; identifies with male and female genders, reflected in gender-neutral dress	Cisgender male (he/him/his) Born biological male; identifies as a man

TABLE 15–1. Examples of power, individual identity, and group membership salience in clinicians *(continued)*

	Clinician 1	Clinician 2	Clinician 3
Regional upbringing	West Coaster Grew up in Los Angeles, California, and is living on the East Coast for the first time	Southerner Grew up in Birmingham, Alabama, and has lived in every region of the United States	New Englander Grew up in Boston, Massachusetts, and has never lived in any other state
Political views	Liberal Ideologically liberal and votes Democrat	Conservative Ideologically conservative but votes Democrat	Libertarian Independent ideologically and votes Independent
Parents' socioeconomic status and education	Upper middle class Both parents attended college	Upper class Both parents have graduate degrees	Lower middle class Both parents have high school diplomas
Hobbies	Sports (soccer)	Electronics (video gaming)	Dance (swing dancing)
Medical specialty	Child and adolescent psyhiatry	Interventional psychiatry	Forensic psychiatry
Personality	Extrovert Outgoing personality Proactively asks for desires	Introvert Shy Reactively asks for desires	Both Shy at work, outgoing at home
Generation	Generation Z	Millennial	Boomer
Preferred mode of communication	Prefers text communication	No preference between text or phone	Prefers telephone or in-person contact

Recognize Injustice and Your Role in Addressing It

When we have increased self and societal awareness, the manifestations of inequity in our professional settings will be more evident. A helpful bridge is the concept of *structural vulnerability*. It captures the physical and emotional toll of inequity over time,; recognizes the patterned impact on specific demographic groups; and is best formulated through the viewpoint of the beneficiary, not the advocate (Quesada et al. 2011). As a brief exercise, reflect on your experiences visiting your local post office, bank, or emergency department. Next, consider your expectations of the service at each institution. Then imagine that you were met with the following outcomes:

- The post office did not deliver your package, ran out of stamps, or unexpectedly closed early
- The local bank required a 7-day wait and charged an exorbitant fee to process your check for deposit
- The wait to be seen by a physician at the emergency department was 8 hours, and no clear follow-up instructions were given on discharge

Although these situations may occur rarely, if ever, for you, such service is the status quo in some communities. The absence of institutional investment and the resulting poor service for certain people in certain neighborhoods is a form of institutionalized oppression. The examples above are fairly circumscribed, but imagine the physical and emotional impact of powerful systems—such as educational, carceral, health care, and child welfare—that are repeat perpetrators of structural violence on individuals, families, and communities. This is structural vulnerability.

Individuals are rendered vulnerable through two main forces. The first is exemplified by unfair exclusion from access to resources, such as an appropriate education or high-quality health care. The exclusion is unfair because it stems from the economic exploitation of one group at the hands of those groups with more power. The second force exerted—the individual internalization of societal narratives of unworthiness—is more abstract but potentially more damaging (Quesada et al. 2011). In the patients we serve, this force may manifest as a symptom of hopelessness after generations of exposure to multifaceted structural oppression. A significant risk for mental health providers who serve in these communities is that the routine nature of this oppression makes it appear normal, immutable even. When this occurs, advocacy will not happen. And when we do not advocate, our assumptions about the ineffectiveness of advocacy (and our ability to advocate) goes unchallenged. In reality, our professional standing is one of privilege; thus, we all have some measure of power. In leveraging our privilege to advocate, we must understand our power relative to other stakeholders (Hunt et al. 2019).

The skillful recognition of injustice requires a commitment to active, ongoing learning that will naturally lead to questions about systemic drivers for issues raised in clinical encounters. At times, the application of our newly attained knowledge may be limited by our own assumptions about the reasons for our patients' experiences. For example, when a patient presents with anxiety, but an exploration of these symptoms raises questions about exploitative housing policies, advocacy is an indicated intervention. This is true regardless of our assumptions about potential individual contributors to the conflict, such as the patient's negative interpersonal interactions with the landlord. The patient's maladaptive coping strategies do not justify clinician inaction when that patient is faced with the potential loss of home. As mental health professionals with knowledge of structural violence and social injustice, we have an ethical duty to aid the patient in conceptualizing, pursuing, and realizing a more just outcome—and a healthier one.

In clinical settings, multiple power dynamics are at play within a given conflict. For example, imagine an early career clinician in the middle of a conflict between a patient and the clinician's supervisor. Before reaching conclusions, the clinician should be intentional about using a structural lens to examine the conflict and all parties' responses. The supervisor not only has the comfort of being in a position of power but also may have an advanced vocabulary and fair affect regulation. As a result, the supervisor readily articulates the conflict with illustrative language and an even-keeled tone. Consequently, understanding the supervisor's perspective requires little effort by the clinician. The patient, however, is at a power disadvantage with both the clinician and the supervisor. Furthermore, for a patient with depressive symptoms and prior experiences with structural trauma, the conflict and power differentials may cause withdrawal and hopelessness. Understanding the patient's perspective will require more work by the clinician, who will have to use active listening, open-ended questions, and patience to allow the patient to adequately express thoughts. Systemic injustice could cloud the supervisor's lens and muffle the patient's voice. In the absence of this understanding, both the supervisor and the clinician will be ill equipped to help the patient. Worse, they could be agents of the patient's oppression.

As we practice recognizing injustice, our knowledge gained translates more readily into the understanding of professional experiences in real time. However, at no point is understanding free from the impact of our

TABLE 15–2. Self-reflection questions

Topic	Questions
System	Am I part of or outside of the affected system?
Social group	Am I part of the privileged group or the oppressed group?
Style	Will I intervene indirectly or confront directly?
Self-view	Do I see myself as personally effective or ineffective?
Information	Do I know a lot or a little? How accurate is what I know?
Consequence	Will the personal and organizational consequences be major or minor?

Source. Hunt et al. 2019.

own biases and power. In recognizing injustice and our role in addressing it, ongoing self-examination is critical. Table 15–2 includes some helpful questions for continuing self-reflection.

Understanding our role in the redistribution of justice requires awareness of stereotypes paired with careful examination of discriminatory actions. Advocates also must be aware of how their status and power influence others and learn how to appropriately analyze this power. For example, imagine that psychiatric residents working on an inpatient unit are debating the impact of trauma on a patient with emotional lability and chronic suicidality in the setting of current domestic violence. After the attending physician makes a single comment and gesture, the entire group's conceptualization of the patient's problem and the nature of her treatment plan could change dramatically. Think of the impact of the following scenarios:

1. The attending rolls his eyes and characterizes the patient as "classic borderline personality disorder."
2. The attending nods his head and identifies the patient's financial dependence on her abusive partner as a barrier to her escape from harm.

Because of the physician's position of authority as an attending physician, his seemingly small comment effectively ends the residents' debate, whether or not that was his intention. In the first scenario, the attending physician's comment could amplify negative countertransference toward the patient, undermine her therapeutic alliance with her treating psychiatrist, and lead to a referral for dialectical behavior therapy. In the second scenario, the attending physician's comment could increase the residents' empathy toward the patient, bolster the therapeutic alliance, and result in her treating psy-

TABLE 15–3. Analysis of power and influence

Throughout the exercise, identify any unfounded beliefs or assumptions about specific identities, be curious about how the belief was formed and shaped, and identify examples of how these beliefs could manifest relationally in various professional settings. Using the identities contained in Table 15–1 as a starting point, apply each question to each professional setting listed below.

Questions

1. As a result of their different identities, how might the clinicians differ in their interactions as mental health professionals?

2. As a result of their different career stages, how might the clinicians differ in their interactions as mental health professionals?

3. As a result of their different combinations of identities, how might the clinicians differ in their interactions as mental health professionals?

4. How might your approach to collaboration on an advocacy project differ in working with each clinician?

5. Looking specifically at the career stage or identities that you align with, how do you perceive these aspects influencing your interactions as a mental health professional?

Professional settings

A. Clinical encounter with a patient in your typical patient population

B. Treatment team meeting with a clinical team whose composition is comparable to the composition of colleagues in your work environment

C. Social event for the entire clinic staff with a composition of clinicians, administrative staff, supervisors, trainees, and other support staff typical of your work environment

chiatrist collaborating with the unit social worker to identify housing resources for battered women. Table 15–3 includes prompts for practicing analysis of power and influence.

Respond to Injustice Through an Iterative, Sustainable Process

In each advocacy effort, the strategy employed will depend on resources possessed by the individual, collaborator, or community; the context, be it within family, health care, or public arenas; and, most importantly, the ad-

vocate's knowledge and power relative to others. Mental health professionals can employ the following three-step process to respond to injustice
strategically and effectively.

Step 1: Explore, Identify, and Assess the Implicit and Explicit Needs of the Patient

Feelings of vulnerability are uncomfortable and may prove difficult to acknowledge. For some individuals, these feelings may be outright triggering
and could result in withdrawal, agitation, or guardedness. Understandably,
patients who feel vulnerable rarely present with spontaneously expressed,
detailed explanations of the detrimental impact of oppression on their lives.
Knowledge gained through study of self and systems provides clinicians
with the requisite context for knowing what to listen for in patients' histories, what questions to ask, and other potential sources of helpful information. Table 15–4 illustrates how this process might be applied to a sample
clinical scenario.

Step 2: Brainstorm Feasible Interventions With the Potential for Discernible Benefits and Tolerable Consequences

After you have identified factors that can be ameliorated by advocacy efforts, the next step is to critically examine individual motives, assumptions,
and insecurities concerning the patient and the context. Then, you must
decide if action is needed and feasible in the *micro* (clinical), *meso* (community), or *macro* (public policy) settings. While evaluating the options for intervention, you should explore possible actions and outcomes
collaboratively with the patient. Then, the goals of and proposed approach
to advocacy must be communicated with the stakeholders who have the
most to lose and the least influence. Obtaining buy-in promotes group cohesion and facilitates collaboration. It is also important to note that feasible
options for advocacy are shaped substantially by the advocates' relationship
to power.

As an example, consider the case of Stan (see Table 15–4), a patient with
worsening mental health symptoms in the context of roommate conflicts in
his group home. Even though an intern, resident, and attending physician
all may recognize this as a key issue, their options for advocacy will differ.

TABLE 15–4. Case example: exploring, identifying, and assessing a patient's implicit and explicit needs

Stan, age 28, is currently living in a sober house. He has had an increase in hospitalizations and emergency department visits since he was assigned a new roommate, who is regularly using substances. Stan has been able to maintain sobriety for the past year in hopes of getting his own apartment. He has been on the waiting list for a housing voucher for 1 year.

Identified patient needs are relief from a distressing roommate dynamic, support during a stressful period that poses a risk to sobriety, and reassuring yet realistic updates about the status of alternative housing.

Potential solutions	Potential benefits	Potential consequences	Uncertainties
Change roommate	Might alleviate acute distress	Missed opportunity to improve coping skills	Are there open rooms in the group home? Do other residents use substances?
Inpatient admission for stabilization	Offers a safe, structured, substance-free environment while symptoms are stabilized	Inability to cope with stressors of unstructured environment	Are there open beds? Does Stan meet criteria for inpatient admission? Where will he go when discharged?
Move Stan up the waiting list	Offers more timely relief from distress of living situation	Missed opportunity to work through frustration from lack of access to resources	Is it possible to move patients up the list? Is the process one that you can influence? Is the housing authority report reliable?

- The intern would have less authority within the institution and be less likely to have established connections across agencies. Given these circumstances, the intern's advocacy options might include motivational interviewing with Stan, calling to ask about open rooms in the group home, or researching activities for him so that his time at the group home can be minimized.
- The resident would have more authority to act independently but would still need approval for major decisions. The resident also may not have authority that translates to other agencies. As such, the resident's

options might include recommending hospitalization to the attending physician or calling the group home manager and asking about the process for switching roommates.

- The attending physician would have greater authority as the top decision maker on the team, as well as by virtue of having established relationships at other agencies. Thus, the attending's options might be calling the group home manager directly to request a roommate change or hospitalizing Stan immediately.

Table 15–5 lists some more specific, concrete approaches to advocacy.

Step 3: Evaluate and Reassess

As with any intervention, assessment of advocacy's effectiveness and shortcomings is necessary for improvement. This task can range from a simple follow-up with the patient about the outcome to a robust data-gathering process. In the same way you as a mental health professional receive supervision and feedback in developing clinical skills, so must you also receive feedback and support in developing your advocacy skills. Improvement can happen only when there is an understanding of how efforts were effective or what needs improvement. It is important to know which strategies are worth repeating and which strategies need to be reformulated. At a minimum, you should actively seek feedback on your advocacy efforts from both patients and collaborators.

Conclusion

Each of us need not be familiar with every advocacy model, competency, or strategy to play a role in the pursuit of social justice. In the service of our patients, many of us already advocate in ways we may not recognize: calling repeatedly to reach an agency supervisor, writing grant proposals for community programs, or connecting a patient with a nearby food pantry. In actuality, advocacy takes place whenever unmet needs are acknowledged and addressed (Marshall-Lee et al. 2019). Building a sustainable, effective, long-term advocacy practice requires engaging both personal and professional supports, appreciating the advocacy that has been accomplished, and seeking ways to improve. Because this work may be met by reactions to defend the status quo, commitment to advocacy requires both moral courage and the collective strength found in solidarity and community support.

TABLE 15–5. Advocacy competencies

Competency	Descriptions of examples
Patient empowerment	Identify patients' strengths and resources
	Recognize the signs indicating that an individual's behaviors and concerns reflect responses to systemic or internalized oppression
	Support patients in developing self-advocacy action skills
	Help patients gain access to needed resources
Patient advocacy	Co-create with patient a plan that includes rationale and possible outcomes of advocacy
	Identify potential allies for confronting the barriers
Community	Develop alliances with groups working for change
	Use effective listening skills to gain an understanding of the group's goals
	Identify and respect the strengths and resources that the group members bring to the process of systemic change
Systems	Identify environmental factors impinging on patients' development
	Provide and interpret data to show the urgency for change
	In collaboration with other stakeholders, develop a vision and plan to guide change and seek out opportunities for implementation
Public information	Prepare written and multimedia materials that provide clear explanations of the role of specific environmental factors in human development
	Disseminate information through a variety of media with diverse audiences
	Identify and collaborate with other professionals who are involved in disseminating public information
Social/political	Distinguish those problems that can best be resolved through social or political action
	With allies, prepare convincing data and rationales for change and lobby legislators and other policy makers
	Maintain open dialogue with communities and patients to ensure that social/political advocacy is consistent with the initial goals

Source. American Counseling Association 2018; Lewis et al. 2003; Ratts and Hutchins 2009.

Questions for Self-Reflection

1. Do I identify with the title of *advocate*? How do my personal and professional identities influence these feelings?
2. What are my preferred methods of learning? How can I use these methods to become more knowledgeable about social injustice?
3. What social justice issues are particularly relevant for the population I serve? Have I been intentional in learning more about these issues? Why or why not? How can I learn more?

References

American Counseling Association: Advocacy Competencies. Alexandria, VA, American Counseling Association, 2018. Available at: www.counseling.org/docs/default-source/competencies/aca-advocacy-competencies-updated-may-2020.pdf?sfvrsn=f410212c_4. Accessed on September 7, 2020.

Chung RC, Bernak F, Talleyrand RM, Williams JM: Challenges in promoting race dialogues in psychology training: race and gender perspectives. Couns Psychol 46:213–240, 2018

Hunt MG, Miller RA, Stacy MA, et al: Public servant, silent servant: a call to action for advocacy training in public service settings. Psychol Serv 2019 Epub ahead of print

Lewis JA, Arnold MS, House R, Toporek RL: Advocacy Competencies. Alexandria, VA, American Counseling Association, 2003. Available at: www.counseling.org/resources/competencies/advocacy_competencies.pdf. Accessed on April 28, 2020

Marshall-Lee ED, Hinger C, Popovic R, et al: Social justice advocacy in mental health services: consumer, community, training, and policy perspectives. Psychol Serv 2019 Epub ahead of print

The Physicians Foundation: Survey of America's Physicians: Practice Patterns and Perspectives. September 18, 2018. Available at: https://physiciansfoundation.org/research-insights/the-physicians-foundation-2018-physician-survey. Accessed January 10, 2020.

Quesada J, Hart LK, Bourgois P: Structural vulnerability and health: Latino migrant laborers in the United States. Med Anthropol 30:339–362, 2011

Ratts MJ, Hutchins AM: ACA advocacy competencies: social justice advocacy at the client/student level. J Couns Dev 87:269–275, 2009

Stege AR, Brockberg D, Hoyt W: Advocating for advocacy: an exploratory survey on student advocacy skills and training in counseling psychology. Train Educ Prof Psychol 11:190–197, 2017

CHAPTER 16

Social Justice and Mental Health

A Call to Action

Sarah Y. Vinson, M.D.
Ruth S. Shim, M.D., M.P.H.

Who doesn't love a feel-good story about someone who beat the odds? There is a reason so many books are filled with such stories. We cheer the heroes' and heroines' grit; we applaud their hard work. And we hold them up as examples for those comparably situated and at risk of becoming a statistic. It is natural to focus on individual narratives, be they courageous inspirations or cautionary tales, but doing so obscures the real story. It is not about the individuals who defied the odds or those who were defined by them; it is about the odds themselves. This book is about the injustice inherent in society's stacked odds—their drivers, their design, and their detrimental impact on society's mental health. It details how social injustice—rather than individuals or cultural factors—is the antagonist in the narrative of the struggle for mental health equity.

Driven by societal perceptions about the inherent worth and value of certain people, our country's laws, policies, and systems are designed to benefit some and harm others. Predictably, the results are inequitable, and the mental health system is no exception. These structures effectively operate as they are designed, replicating social hierarchies and oppression with no need for our active awareness or conscious contribution. A neutral stance is a complicit one, enabling the status quo and the inequities that come with it. The active stance required to dismantle these structures and systems will require significant effort.

Before asking more of you, however, we must first acknowledge the work you have already done. Simply by engaging with this text, you have confronted the hard truths contained herein, overcome your defenses to sincerely self-reflect, and, hopefully, increased your awareness and understanding of social injustice in mental health. As coeditors of this book, we cheer your perseverance, applaud your work, and are immensely grateful for your time. If you have not already done so, take a moment to reflect on the truths you have already uncovered, the commitments you have already made, and the action you have already taken. And when you are ready, get back to work. Hopefully, this experience surpasses increased knowledge, extending to greater resolve and commitment to the pursuit of social justice in order to achieve mental health equity. We all have more to learn, and we all have more to do. As we focus on the odds themselves, critically examining our field and the larger society, the sheer scope of injustice and its myriad manifestations may elicit hopelessness and despondency. But we cannot yield to these inclinations. In the words of singer and activist Joan Baez, "Action is the antidote to despair" (Loder 1983). Each of us has the power to act. *And the time to begin is now.*

Achieving Mental Health Equity

Part I of this book provides a framework for thinking about why mental health inequities exist and persist and about the structural drivers of these inequities. In *The Wretched of the Earth*, psychiatrist Frantz Fanon (2004, p. 236) wrote that "we need a model, schemas, and examples" that are different from our traditional inherited European models based in oppression and othering. To truly achieve mental health equity, we must consider different models, schemas, and examples in the way we think about and examine social injustice in mental health.

Education and Training

To counter the powerful forces of social injustice in mental health, we must transform existing societal structures. This effort begins with mental health education and training. Mental health professional and medical education training impart knowledge of psychology, psychiatry, and psychopathology. Although this knowledge is necessary, it is not enough. As discussed in Chapter 15, "Social Justice and Advocacy," change requires adopting an active practice of self-study and self-reflection. Building on the foundation of the content in this book, Table 16–1 provides a starting point—it is by no means a definitive list—of supplemental learning materials. This resource list should function as a living document and is intended to be added to and updated regularly.

Additionally, knowledge of social justice and mental health equity should be infused into formal education and training at all levels. Many undergraduate and graduate schools, medical schools, nursing schools, certificate programs, and residency programs are beginning to recognize the importance of social justice education in mental health. Some are fortunate to have expert faculty and instructors to guide students and facilitate effective learning. However, many educational programs struggle to identify faculty and instructors with structural and social justice expertise in their learning communities. In reality, a treasure trove of untapped knowledge is at most educators' fingertips. Many patients, community members, students, and trainees possess deep expertise in social justice issues. It is our biased ideas of who are *experts* that prevent us from accessing this wisdom. Policies blindly reliant on educational standards often create barriers that prevent experts with less formal training from imparting valuable knowledge to students and trainees. Furthermore, when these experts are asked to teach, they are often expected to volunteer and are not appropriately compensated for their time and expertise.

Therefore, focusing on policy change to promote this type of interdisciplinary education is worthwhile. Education and curricula around social justice should be driven and directed by those with direct and intimate knowledge of the issues. Growing numbers of graduate and postgraduate students have received extensive training on the foundational disciplines of this work during their undergraduate educations. Students and residents have successfully designed effective social justice and mental health curricula in medical school and residency training settings (Coria et al. 2013; Hixon et al. 2013). Programs such as In Our Own Voice, a series of presentations by the National Alliance on Mental Illness (www.nami.org/Support-Education/Mental-Health-Education/NAMI-In-Our-Own-Voice), provide access to trained speakers with lived experiences seeking and utilizing mental health care services. Experts are among us, but we must have the humility to recognize them and ask for their guidance and insight. Doing so requires recognition that our traditional hierarchies are faulty and that many *less educated* people—or rather, people who are *less schooled*—hold the vast expertise and knowledge required for our profession's progress and promotion.

TABLE 16–1. Social injustice and mental health:
self-study resources

Books

An African American and Latinx History of the United States, Paul Ortiz (2018)

Between the World and Me, Ta-Nehisi Coates (2015)

Black Picket Fences: Privilege and Peril Among the Black Middle Class, Mary Patillo-McCoy (1999)

Black Skin, White Masks, Frantz Fanon (1952/2008 [updated language for new generation of readers])

Caste: The Origins of Our Discontents, Isabel Wilkerson (2020)

The Color of Law: Our Forgotten History of How Our Government Segregated America, Richard Rothstein (2017)

The Deepest Well: Healing the Long-Term Effects of Childhood Adversity, Nadine Burke Harris (2018)

A Disability History of the United States, Kim E. Nielson (2012)

Evicted: Poverty and Profit in the American City, Matthew Desmond (2016)

Fatal Invention: How Science, Politics, and Big Business Re-create Race in the Twenty-First Century, Dorothy Roberts (2011)

Freedom is a Constant Struggle: Ferguson, Palestine, and the Foundations of a Movement, Angela Y. Davis (2016)

Ghetto Schooling: A Political Economy of Urban Educational Reform, Jean Anyon (1997)

High Price: A Neuroscientist's Journey of Self-Discovery That Challenges Everything You Know About Drugs and Society, Carl Hart (2013)

Hillbilly Elegy: A Memoir of a Family and Culture in Crisis, J.D. Vance (2016)

The History of White People, Nell Irvin Painter (2011)

Hood Feminism, Mikki Kendall (2020)

How to Be Antiracist, Ibram X. Kendi (2019)

Immigrant America: A Portrait, Alejandro Portes and Rubén G. Rumbaut (1990)

An Indigenous Peoples' History of the United States, Roxanne Dunbar-Ortiz (2014)

Lies My Teacher Told Me: Everything Your American History Textbooks Got Wrong, James W. Loewen (1995)

Medical Apartheid: The Dark History of Medical Experimentation on Black Americans From Colonial Times to the Present, Harriet A. Washington (2007)

TABLE 16–1. Social injustice and mental health: self-study resources *(continued)*

Books *(continued)*

The New Jim Crow: Mass Incarceration in the Age of Colorblindness, Michelle Alexander (2010)

The Origin of Others, Toni Morrison (2017)

Pedagogy of the Oppressed, 30th Anniversary Edition, Paulo Freire (2000)

A People's History of the United States, Howard Zinn (1980)

People's Science: Bodies and Rights on the Stem Cell Frontier, Ruha Benjamin (2013)

The Protest Psychosis: How Schizophrenia Became a Black Disease, Jonathan Metzl (2009)

Pushout: The Criminalization of Black Girls in Schools, Monique W. Morris (2015)

Queer (In)Justice: The Criminalization of LGBT People in the United States, Joey L. Mogul, Andrea J. Ritchie, and Kay Whitlock (2012)

Racism Without Racists: Color-Blind Racism and the Persistence of Racial Inequality in America, Eduardo Bonilla-Silva (2003)

Root Shock: How Tearing Up City Neighborhoods Hurts America, and What We Can Do About It, Mindy Thompson Fullilove (2004)

Savage Inequalities: Children in America's Schools, Jonathan Kozol (1991)

The Second Sex, Simone De Beauvoir, translated by Constance Borde and Sheila Malovany-Chevallier (1949/2011)

Sister Outsider: Essays and Speeches (1984)

Stamped From the Beginning: The Definitive History of Racist Ideas in America, Ibram X. Kendi (2016)

Structural Competency in Mental Health and Medicine: A Case-Based Approach to Treating the Social Determinants of Health, Helena Hansen and Jonathan M. Metzl (2019)

Trauma and Recovery—The Aftermath of Violence—From Domestic Abuse to Political Terror, Judith Herman (1992)

The Warmth of Other Suns: The Epic Story of America's Great Migration, Isabel Wilkerson (2011)

We Should All Be Feminists, Chimamanda Ngozi Adichie (2014)

White Fragility: Why It's So Hard for White People to Talk About Racism, Robin DiAngelo (2018)

Why Are All the Black Kids Sitting Together in the Cafeteria?: And Other Conversations About Race (20th Anniversary Edition), Beverly Daniel Tatum (2017)

TABLE 16–1. Social injustice and mental health:
                      self-study resources *(continued)*

Documentaries

American Factory, Steven Bognar and Julia Reichert (2019)

The Death and Life of Marsha P. Johnson, David France (2017)

Harlan County, USA, Barbara Kopple (1977)

The House I Live In, Eugene Jarecki (2017)

The Hunting Ground, Kirby Dick (2015)

I Am Not Your Negro, Raoul Peck (2017)

Immigration Nation, Christina Clusiau and Shaul Schwarz (2020)

The New Asylums, Miri Navasky and Karen O'Connor (2005)

Out in the Night, Blair Dorosh-Walther (2014)

Paper Tigers, James Redford (2015)

A Place at the Table, Lori Silverbush and Kristi Jacobson (2012)

13th, Ava Duvernay (2016)

Time to Choose, Charles Ferguson (2015)

Unnatural Causes: Is Inequality Making Us Sick?, California Newsreel (2018)

Podcasts

About Race With Reni Eddo-Lodge

Code Switch

The Diversity Gap

Intersectionality Matters With Kimberlé Crenshaw

Seeing White

Serial—Season 3

The 1619 Podcast

Ted talks

"America's Forgotten Working Class," J.D. Vance

"The Danger of a Single Story," Chimamanda Ngozi Adichie

"How Childhood Trauma Affects Health Across a Lifetime," Nadine Burke Harris

"How Does Income Affect Childhood Brain Development?" Kimberly Noble

"How Economic Inequality Harms Societies," Richard Wilkinson

TABLE 16–1. Social injustice and mental health: self-study resources *(continued)*

Ted talks *(continued)*

"How We're Priming Some Kids for College—and Others for Prison," Alice Goffman

"Our Fight for Disability Rights, and Why We're Not Done Yet," Judith Heumann

"A Prosecutor's Vision for a Better Justice System," Adam Foss

"To Transform Child Welfare, Take Race Out of the Equation," Jessica Pryce

"The Urgency of Intersectionality," Kimberlé Crenshaw

"We Need to Talk About an Injustice," Bryan Stevenson

"What If Gentrification Was About Healing Communities Instead of Harming Them?" Liz Ogbu

Research

As discussed in Chapter 14, "Social Justice and Mental Health System Reform," academic research has traditionally prioritized the needs of the institution over the participants and communities being studied. These communities, while adjacent to economically powerful academic institutions, are often plagued by oppression and divestment. Additionally, many researchers, who are well-meaning and committed to examining and reducing mental health inequities, design and conduct their research with a focus on identifying individual-level differences. As a result, they often fail to consider the structural context that shapes (or explains) these differential outcomes. For example, at the foundational level, many researchers do not acknowledge the gross imprecision of using race as a variable. Demographic data on race are often gathered and interpreted without an understanding of the principles discussed in Chapter 3, "Social Injustice and Mental Health Inequities," and Chapter 4, "Social Injustice and Structural Racism." Researchers often fail to understand that race is socially constructed and is most often a rough, inexact proxy for many other factors, including social status, geography, culture, and genetics. This omission leads to dangerous misattributions and inaccuracies in research, including reinforcement of biological determinism and negative biases (Chowkwanyun and Reed 2020). This problem is evident in examining current research on health inequities of Asian American populations, in which multiple, extremely diverse subgroups are lumped together and reported in aggregate, rendering invalid any of the conclusions drawn from this aggregated data (Gordon et al. 2019).

Just as researchers must complete mandatory training in basic ethical principles, as stated in the Belmont Report (National Commission for the Protection of Human Subjects of Biomedical and Behavioral Research 1979), so, too, should they be required to complete training in racism, sexism, and implicit bias. Additionally, they should learn about methods of conducting research and approaches to interpreting results that avoid the perpetuation of structural violence and social injustice. Similarly, peer-reviewed journals must prioritize recruiting clinicians and scientists from backgrounds underrepresented in mental health and medicine to serve on editorial boards (Kennedy et al. 2001). They must also employ experts in implicit bias and mental health inequities to provide effective peer review so that the dissemination of problematic data collection and interpretation is prevented. In academic settings, many mental health professionals have the power to call attention to these issues and to lead in the implementation of these needed changes.

The goal of social justice–informed education and research would also be furthered by reexamining the selection and leadership development process in training and academic institutions. In the mentoring, sponsoring, hiring, and vetting processes, it is natural that those in positions of power (attending physicians, supervisors, training directors, department and division chairs, admissions committees, and search committee members) will be susceptible to affinity bias and overvalue their own networks and contacts. This means that in the absence of corrective action, the demographics of mental health professionals considered for opportunities (through graduate or medical school admission, inclusion in abstracts or research papers, or interviews for leadership positions) will mirror those of the current decision makers. Furthermore, aspiring and practicing mental health professionals with valuable experientially based perspectives on social injustice have been subjected to structural barriers throughout their educational process, decreasing the utility of apples-to-apples comparisons of academic credentials. Consideration of these issues makes the case for holistic review of applicants across all levels of education, training, and careers. These issues also necessitate the deliberate, systematic consideration and inclusion of people from underrepresented groups in mentorship programs, scholarly activity, and searches for institutional leaders.

Social Injustice and Systems

As discussed in Part II of this book, the many systems that structure our society often perpetuate social injustice. To treat or cure the mental health problems caused and sustained by these systems, we must change the laws and policies that govern them. Accomplishing such change requires that we take political stances, which can make many people uncomfortable. We acknowledge (and understand) that for many it is more palatable to take a politically neutral stance, especially in the current political environment in which Americans are seemingly more politically divided than ever. However, remaining apolitical, or neutral, *is* a political stance. It is a tacit acceptance of the status quo. Mental health equity should be an aspiration of all professionals committed to addressing mental illness. It need not be a partisan issue. We have a collective responsibility to promote policies that make our structures more just and, as a result, our mental health outcomes more equitable. With an understanding of the social determinants of mental health, it becomes clear that all policies have health and mental health impacts. Thus, we must interface directly with voters, leaders, policy makers, and local governments to ensure that *all* policies promote equity and neither sustain nor exacerbate oppression or structural violence. This undertaking also requires interfacing with communities and forming cross-sector collaborations to intentionally bring marginalized communities to the table. As pathologist and politician Rudolf Virchow said, "Medicine is a social science, and politics is nothing else but medicine on a large scale" (Friedlander 2005).

Mental Health Diagnoses and Conditions

In Part III of this book, we examine specific mental health diagnoses and conditions through a social justice lens. Many of us are clinicians and spend much of our time doing clinical work. Thus, it is important to consider effective interventions that can infuse principles of social justice into our clinical settings.

Clinical Practice

As discussed in Chapter 2, "Social Injustice and the Social Determinants of Mental Health," a "preferential option for the poor" requires that mental health professionals adjust their frame of reference and err on the side of doing more for disadvantaged patients. We can do this at the policy and procedural level of clinical practice by thinking about how our clinical settings operate. In taking a deliberate, data-driven approach to analyzing existing policies to see if they create barriers to care for some patients, we take the first step in addressing those barriers. We can also do this work in individual clinical encounters by listening more intently and giving the benefit of the doubt more quickly to those who have experienced more oppression and othering.

An important strategy for infusing social justice into clinical practice is that of *accompaniment*, or the process of trying to minimize power dynamics in clinical relationships by listening, witnessing, and advocating with patients. Often, when our patients are nonadherent to our treatment recommendations, we experience a range of emotions, including disappointment, frustration, and anger. These are certainly valid emotions, but we can repurpose them as a useful signal reminding us to consider ways that we might *walk alongside* our patients, to seek greater understanding of their personal experiences influencing their nonadherent behaviors (Watkins 2015). The medical concept of shared decision making is movement in this direction, but the work of accompaniment requires mental health professionals to practice radical empathy. Within the mental health professions, peer specialists skillfully and routinely practice accompaniment, and mental health professionals of all backgrounds can observe and learn how to develop this skill and more effectively incorporate it into practice.

Negative Workers

The term *negative workers* was created by sociologist René Lorau and expanded on by psychiatrist Franco Basaglia and anthropologist Nancy Scheper-Hughes (Watkins 2015). Negative workers are professionals who give their allegiance to those who are most in need, over and above the institutions to which they are employed. Scheper-Hughes (1995) describes the negative worker as "a species of class traitor—a doctor, a teacher, a lawyer, psychologist, a social worker, a manager, a social scientist, even—who colludes with the powerless to identify their needs against the interests of the bourgeois institution: the university, the hospital, the factory" (p. 420). Armed with the knowledge of social injustice in the mental health profession, a growing number of negative mental health workers—strategically located in various institutions and systems throughout the United States—could spark a significant shift toward mental health equity.

A Call to Action

We are aware that substantive barriers to this work exist. That said, many barriers are attributable to distortions in our internal and societal schemas. The broader narratives of American exceptionalism and rugged individualism cloud our view of society's inequities and run counter to structural remedies for addressing them. The Pledge of Allegiance of the United States describes a land of "liberty and justice for all." These words were untrue at our nation's inception, at the time the pledge was written, and at the time of this book's printing. Yet this narrative—that all Americans have success within their reach if they only work hard enough—persists and does so to the nation's detriment. It provides cover for the poor to be exploited by the rich, a rationale for people deemed less deserving to be left behind by policies, and an impetus for public health principles to be pitted against individual rights and calls for self-determination.

The progress you make in your appreciation of the nature of these distortions and the scope of their harmful impact may surpass that of those around you. Resistance to this effort is inevitable. When progress *is* made, as has happened many times throughout history, we tend to breathe a sigh of relief and celebrate. We are not always prepared for the inevitable retrenchment that accompanies progress (The Aspen Institute 2016). As we prepare to do the work, we must strategize and plan for this. If we fail to prepare for retrenchment, its sheer force can be demoralizing. As civil rights leader and congressman John Lewis said, "Do not get lost in a sea of despair. Be hopeful, be optimistic. Our struggle is not the struggle of a day, a week, a month, or a year, it is the struggle of a lifetime. Never, ever be afraid to make some noise and get in good trouble, necessary trouble" (Bote 2020).

If you are successful at this task, at times your gains, and sometimes even you personally, will be undermined. There is no doubt that the work ahead is hard. But our profession, our patients, and our society need us, and they need us for years to come. This work must be done sustainably, and self-care is a prerequisite. The great writer and activist Audre Lorde once said, "Caring for myself is not self-indulgence, it is self-preservation, and that is an act of political warfare" (Lorde 1988, p. 130). Self-care is essential for the work of social justice. It enables us to advocate for others—amplifying our effectiveness and extending our time. Many of us know what works for us as individuals, but we simply have not decided to prioritize it. Incorporating what works into your routine and fiercely protecting it is critical. Furthermore, this personal self-care practice must be bolstered through investment in meaningful personal and professional connections, allowing you to tap into the strength found in community.

Conclusion

> Life is very short, and what we have to do must be done in the now.
>
> *Audre Lorde (Hall 2004, p. 72)*

If, after reading this book, you are not up for joining the fight for social justice in mental health, we appreciate your openness. We are grateful that you read it anyway. If you were part of the fight for social justice in mental health *before* reading this book, we hope you found it helpful. We continue to be inspired and supported by your energy and commitment. If you are up for joining the fight for social justice *after* reading this book, we are thrilled. We welcome you and look forward to our future collaborations. There is much work to be done. Our patients deserve—and are entitled to—the opportunity to live their lives in a world in which good mental health is within everyone's reach.

Questions for Self-Reflection

1. How has my understanding of social injustice and mental health changed as a result of reading this book?
2. How can I grow my knowledge of social justice in ways that fit my learning style? What commitments am I willing to make toward acquiring this knowledge?
3. What are some ways that I can apply social justice principles in my current personal and professional communities?

References

The Aspen Institute: Racial Equity: 11 Terms You Should Know to Better Understand Structural Racism. Washington, DC, Aspen Institute, July 11, 2016. Available at: www.aspeninstitute.org/blog-posts/structural-racism-definition. Accessed May 15, 2020.

Bote J: 'Get in good trouble, necessary trouble': Rep. John Lewis in his own words. USA Today, July 19, 2020. Available at: www.usatoday.com/story/news/politics/2020/07/18/rep-john-lewis-mostmemorable-quotes-get-good-trouble/5464148002. Accessed September 4, 2020

Coria A, McKelvey TG, Charlton P, et al: The design of a medical school social justice curriculum. Acad Med 88:1442–1449, 2013

Chowkwanyun M, Reed AL Jr: Racial health disparities and COVID-19: caution and context. N Engl J Med 383(3):201–203, 2020 Epub ahead of print

Fanon F: The Wretched of the Earth. New York, Grove Press, 2004

Friedlander E: Rudolf Virchow on pathology education. Presented at the Meeting of the Group for Research in Pathology Education, Hershey, PA, January 30, 2005. Available at: www.pathguy.com/virchow.htm. Accessed September 7, 2020.

Gordon NP, Lin TY, Rau J, Lo JC: Aggregation of Asian-American subgroups masks meaningful differences in health and health risks among Asian ethnicities: an electronic health record based cohort study. BMC Public Health 19(1):1551–1565, 2019

Hall JW (ed): Conversations With Audre Lorde. Literary Conversations Series. Jackson, University Press of Mississippi, 2004

Hixon AL, Yamada S, Farmer PE, Maskarinec GG: Social justice: the heart of medical education. Soc Med 7:161–168, 2013

Kennedy BL, Lin Y, Dickstein LJ: Women on the editorial boards of major journals. Acad Med 76:849–851, 2001

Loder K: Joan Baez: The Rolling Stone Interview. Rolling Stone, April 14, 1983. Available at: www.rollingstone.com/music/music-features/joan-baez-the-rolling-stone-interview-71113. Accessed September 4, 2020

Lorde A: A Burst of Light and Other Essays. Ithaca, NY, Firebrand Books, 1988

National Commission for the Protection of Human Subjects of Biomedical and Behavioral Research: The Belmont Report. Washington, DC, Office of the Secretary, April 18, 1979. Available at: www.hhs.gov/ohrp/sites/default/files/the-belmont-report-508c_FINAL.pdf. Accessed September 7, 2020.

Scheper-Hughes N: The primacy of the ethical: propositions for a militant anthropology. Curr Anthropol 36:409–440, 1995

Watkins M: Psychosocial accompaniment. Journal of Social and Political Psychology 3:324–341, 2015

Index

Page numbers printed in **boldface** type refer to tables or figures.